Public Health: Practices, Methods and Policies

Professor Joav Merrick, MD, MMedSci, DMSc (Series Editor)
National Institute of Child Health and Human Development, Jerusalem, Israel

"Public Health" is a book series with publications from a multidisciplinary group of researchers, practitioners and clinicians for an international professional forum interested in the broad spectrum of public health issues.

About the Editor-in-Chief
Joav Merrick, MD, MMedSci, DMSc, born and educated in Denmark is Professor of Pediatrics affiliated with the Division of Pediatrics, Hadassah Hebrew University Medical Center, Mt Scopus Campus, Jerusalem, Israel, Kentucky Children's Hospital, University of Kentucky, Lexington, United States and Professor of Public Health at the Center for Healthy Development, School of Public Health, Georgia State University, Atlanta, United States, the former medical director of the Disability Administration, Ministry of Social Affairs and Social Services, Jerusalem and the founder and director of the National Institute of Child Health and Human Development in Israel. Email: jmerrick@zahav.net.il

nova
Medicine & Health
New York

Public Health: Practices, Methods and Policies

Public Health: Implications of Health Behaviors and Diseases
Emmanuel O. Keku, MD, MA, MSPH (Editor)
Joav Merrick, MD, MMedSci, DMSc (Editor)
2023. ISBN: 979-8-89113-083-8 (Hardcover)
2023. ISBN: 979-8-89113-232-0 (eBook)

Positive Youth Development: The Tin Ka Ping P.A.T.H.S. Project in Mainland China
Daniel T.L. Shek, PhD, FHKPS, BBS, SBS, (Editor)
Moon YM Law, RSW, MSW, (Editor)
Xiaoqin Zhu, (Editor)
Joav Merrick, MD, MMedSci, DMSc (Editor)
2022. ISBN: 979-8-88697-282-5 (Softcover)
2022. ISBN: 979-8-88697-324-2 (eBook)

Public Health: Recent International Research
Joav Merrick, MD, MMedSci, DMSc (Editor), Mohammed Morad, MD (Editor)
2022. ISBN: 978-1-68507-491-3 (Hardcover)
2022. ISBN: 978-1-68507-638-2 (eBook)

Environmental Justice and the Intersection of Poverty, Racism and Child Health Disparities
I. Leslie Rubin, MD (Editor), Joav Merrick, MD, MMedSci, DMSc (Editor)
2022. ISBN: 978-1-68507-489-0 (Hardcover)
2022. ISBN: 978-1-68507-640-5 (eBook)

Science, Culture, and Politics: Despair and Hope in the Time of a Pandemic
Consolato M. Sergi, MD (Author)
2021. ISBN: 978-1-53619-816-4 (Hardcover)
2021. ISBN: 978-1-68507-161-5 (eBook)

More information about this series can be found at https://novapublishers.com/product-category/series/public-health-practices-methods-and-policies/

Joav Merrick
Editor

Non-Communicable Diseases

Risk Factors in Lower Income Countries

nova
Medicine & Health
New York

https://doi.org/10.52305/TWAE5031

NOTICE TO THE READER

Library of Congress Cataloging-in-Publication Data

ISBN: 979-8-89113-514-7

Published by Nova Science Publishers, Inc. † New York

Contents

Introduction

Chapter 1

Developmental issues of non-communicable diseases risk factors in lower income countries

Joav Merrick[1-4,*], MD, MMedSci, DMSc
[1]National Institute of Child Health and Human Development, Jerusalem, Israel
[2]Department of Pediatrics, Mt Scopus Campus, Hadassah Hebrew University Medical Center, Jerusalem, Israel
[3]Kentucky Children's Hospital, University of Kentucky, Lexington, Kentucky, United States of America
[4]Center for Healthy Development, School of Public Health, Georgia State University, Atlanta, United States of America

Abstract

Heart disease, stroke, cancer, chronic respiratory diseases and diabetes can be described as non-communicable diseases and are now some of the leading causes of mortality around the world. These diseases result in huge burdens not only for the families involved, but also for society. In this book you will find information and discussion on cervical cancer screening, oral health status, intention to quit smoking, biological and behavioural NCD risk factors, yoga practice, low physical activity, dental service utilisation, dyslipidaemia, sedentary behaviour, soft drink consumption, non-work participation, undiagnosed type 2 diabetes, and undiagnosed, diagnosed and total hypertension in ten countries including Afghanistan, Bangladesh, Bhutan, Bolivia, Ecuador, Eswatini, India, Jordan, Myanmar, and Tonga. It is hoped that findings from these papers may aid public policy and programmes for the prevention and control of non-communicable disease risk factors in lower income countries.

---

* ***Correspondence:*** Professor Joav Merrick, MD, MMedSci, DMSc, Director, National Institute of Child Health and Human Development, Jerusalem, Israel.
Email: jmerrick@zahav.net.il.

In: Non-Communicable Diseases
Editor: Joav Merrick
ISBN: 979-8-89113-514-7

Introduction

"Noncommunicable diseases (NCDs), such as heart disease, stroke, cancer, chronic respiratory diseases and diabetes, are the leading cause of mortality in the world. This invisible epidemic is an under-appreciated cause of poverty and hinders the economic development of many countries. The burden is growing – the number of people, families and communities afflicted is increasing. Common, modifiable risk factors underlie the major NCDs. They include tobacco, harmful use of alcohol, unhealthy diet, insufficient physical activity, overweight/obesity, raised blood pressure, raised blood sugar and raised cholesterol. The NCD threat can be overcome using existing knowledge. The solutions are highly cost-effective. Comprehensive and integrated action at country level, led by governments, is the means to achieve success" (1).

The World Health Organisation (WHO) STEPwise approach to NCD risk factor surveillance (STEPS) is a simple, standardized method for collecting, analysing and disseminating data on key NCD risk factors in countries. The survey instrument covers key behavioural risk factors: tobacco use, alcohol use, physical inactivity, unhealthy diet, as well as key biological risk factors: overweight and obesity, raised blood pressure, raised blood glucose, and abnormal blood lipids. Through the use of expanded modules, the survey instrument can be expanded to cover a range of topics beyond these risk factors, such as oral health, sexual health and road safety" (2).

In this book we discuss cervical cancer screening, oral health status, intention to quit smoking, biological and behavioural NCD risk factors, yoga practice, low physical activity, dental service utilisation, dyslipidaemia, sedentary behaviour, soft drink consumption, non-work participation, undiagnosed type 2 diabetes, and undiagnosed, diagnosed and total hypertension in ten countries including Afghanistan, Bangladesh, Bhutan, Bolivia, Ecuador, Eswatini, India, Jordan, Myanmar, and Tonga. It is hoped that findings from these papers may aid public policy and programmes for the prevention and control of NCD risk factors in lower income countries.

References

[1] World Health Organization. Non-communicable diseases, 2022. URL: https://www.who.int/data/gho/data/themes/noncommunicable-diseases.

[2] World Health Organisation. STEPwise approach to NCD risk factor surveillance (STEPS), 2022. URL: https://www.who.int/teams/noncommunicable-diseases/surveillance/systems-tools/steps.

Section one: International aspects

Chapter 2

Predisposing, enabling and need factors for cervical cancer screening among a national sample of women in Bangladesh

Chao Zhang[1], MD
and Karl Peltzer[2,3,*], PhD

[1]Department of Bone and Soft Tissue Tumors, Tianjin Medical University Cancer Institute and Hospital, National Clinical Research Center for Cancer, Key Laboratory of Cancer Prevention and Therapy, Tianjin's Clinical Research Center for Cancer, Tianjin, China
[2]Department of Psychology, University of the Free State, Bloemfontein, South Africa
[3]Department of Psychology, College of Medical and Health Science, Asia University, Taichung, Taiwan

Abstract

The aim of this chapter was to assess predisposing, enabling and need factors for cervical cancer screening (CCS) among women in Bangladesh. National cross-sectional data were analysed from 2,441 women (30-49 years) who participated in the 2018 Bangladesh STEPS survey. The results show that 6.1% of women ever had undergone CCS. In adjusted logistic regression analysis, health care provider visit in the past 12 months (AOR: 1.78, 95% CI: 1.12-1.82), and having secondary or higher education (AOR: 3.24, 95% CI: 1.60, 6.56), were positively associated with ever having had CCS. In addition, in an unadjusted analysis, urban residence, having diabetes, and central obesity increased

* ***Correspondence:*** Karl Peltzer, Department of Psychology, College of Medical and Health Science, Asia University, Wufeng, Taichung 41354, Taiwan;
Email: kfpeltzer@gmail.com.

In: Non-Communicable Diseases
Editor: Joav Merrick
ISBN: 979-8-89113-514-7

the odds of CCS. The study showed that only one in sixteen women ever had CCS, and several associated factors were found that can be targeted to promote CCS in Bangladesh.

Introduction

Globally, among women cervical cancer (CC) ranks as the fourth highest (1), and among women in Bangladesh it is the second highest (2). "Bangladesh has high burden of CC due to the high prevalence of risk factors like early marriage, early initiation of sexual activity, multiparity, sexually transmitted diseases (STDs) and low socio-economic condition" (2). If CC is diagnosed at an early stage, CC can be successfully treated, which emphasises the need for CC screening (3). In local population-based surveys among women in Bangladesh, for example, in Dhaka, 26% had CCS (4) and in a survey in seven districts in Bangladesh 8.3% of women (30-59 years) had ever CCS (5). Data from 55 low- and middle-income countries (LMICs) showed that among women aged 30-49 years, the median life-time prevalence of CCS was 44% (6). However, we could not find national population-based data on CCS among women in Bangladesh.

Factors associated with CCS may include predisposing factors (such as age and marital status), enabling/disabling factors (access to health care, urban residence, higher socioeconomic status, and positive lifestyle behaviours) and need factors (such as having chronic conditions, obesity, and poor self-rated health status) (6-8). The aim of the study was to assess predisposing, enabling and need factors of CCS among women in Bangladesh. Identifying predictors of CCS may help in CCS promotion planning.

Our study

Cross-sectional national data from the 2018 Bangladesh STEPS survey (9) were analysed; the overall study response rate was 84.6% (10). According to the STEPS survey procedures:

> "Socio-demographic and behavioural information was collected in Step 1. Physical measurements such as height, weight, and blood pressure were collected in Step 2. Biochemical measurements were collected to assess blood glucose and cholesterol levels in Step 3. A multi-stage stratified

> sampling process was carried out to randomly select participants from the target population. One individual within the age range of the survey (18-69 years) was selected per household. Ethics approval was provided by the Bangladesh Medical Research Council (BMRC) and written, or finger impressions (from illiterate participants) informed consent was obtained from all participants" (9, 10).

Data collection followed the "WHO three STEPS methodology: step 1 included administration of a structured questionnaire (sociodemographic, medical history, and health risk behaviour) step 2 consisted of blood pressure and anthropometric measurements, and step 3 included biochemical tests (blood glucose and blood lipids)" (9). Anthropometric measurements were taken using the "Somatometre-Stanley 04-116 device and electronic scales GIMA") (10). Of the three blood pressure measurements using "OMRON Model M5 automatic blood pressure monitor," (10) the last two readings were averaged (9). Five ml of venous blood was collected by "disposable syringe, two ml of this blood was transferred to a fluoride-oxalate vacutainer (brown top) for serum glucose testing and three ml of the blood was kept in a normal tube and allowed to stand for plasma separation (for lipid profile)" (10).

Measures

CCS was asked with the introduction:

> "The next questions I will ask about cervical cancer prevention. Screening tests for cervical cancer prevention can be done in different ways, including visual inspection with acetic acid/vinegar (VIA), pap smear and human papillomavirus (HPV) test. VIA is an inspection of the surface of the uterine cervix after acetic acid (or vinegar) has been applied to it. For both pap smear and HPV test, a doctor or nurse uses a swab to wipe from inside your vagina, take a sample and send it to a laboratory. It is even possible that you were given the swab yourself and asked to swab the inside of your vagina. The laboratory checks for abnormal cell changes if a pap smear is done and for the HP virus if an HPV test is done." And the question was, "Have you ever had a screening test for cervical cancer, using any of these methods described above?" ("Yes, No") (10).

Other questions for those answered with "yes" on CCS included: "When was your last (most recent) test for cervical cancer?" (Responses ranged from "1 = Less than 1 year ago" to "4 = More than 5 years ago); "What is the main reason you had your last test for cervical cancer?" "Where did you receive your last test for cervical cancer?" "What was the result of your last (most recent) test for cervical cancer?" (10).

Predisposing factor questions included marital status, work status, and religion.

Enabling or disabling factor questions included residence status, health care visit in the past 12 months, education, current smokeless tobacco use, fruit and vegetable intake and low physical activity was assessed with the "Global Physical Activity Questionnaire" (11).

Need factors included measured central obesity ("waist circumference ≥90 cm in men, ≥80 cm in women") (12); Hypertension/raised blood pressure (BP): "systolic BP ≥140 mm Hg and/or diastolic BP ≥90 mm Hg or where the participant is currently on antihypertensive medication." (13) Diabetes: "fasting plasma glucose levels >=7.0 mmol/L (≥126 mg/dl); or using insulin or oral hypoglycaemic drugs" (14). Dyslipidaemia was classified (15) as:

> "Being on antilipidemic medication or having one or more of the following: elevated total cholesterol (TC): ≥5.17 mmol/l (200 mg/dl), high triglycerides (TG): ≥1.70 mmol/l (150 mg/dl), low HDL-C: female ≤1.29 mmol/l; ≤male 1.03 (<50 mg/dl in women, <40 mg/dl in men) and high LDL-C: ≥3.36 mmol/l (130 mg/dl)."

History of cardiovascular diseases was assessed with the question "Have you ever had a heart attack or chest pain from heart disease (angina) or a stroke (cerebrovascular accident or incident)?" (Yes/No)

Descriptive statistics were used to summarize the characteristics of the sample and CCS prevalence. Since the World Health Organization recommends CCS for the age group of 30-49 years (16), we restricted the sample for analysis to women aged 30-49 years in our paper. Univariable and multivariable (including variables significant at univariable analysis) logistic regression was used to predict CCS prevalence. Missing values were excluded and $p < 0.05$ was considered significant. Statistical analyses were done with STATA software version 14.0 (Stata Corporation, College Station, TX, USA), taking the complex study design into account.

Table 1. Sample characteristics of women aged 30-49 years, Bangladesh 2018

Variable	Sub-category	Sample	Ever cervical cancer screening
		N (%)	N (%)
All		2441	182 (6.1)
Predisposing factors			
Marital status	Not married Married	156 (5.2) 2285 (94.8)	9 (5.8) 173 (6.1)
Work status	Not employed Employed	2096 (87.6) 339 (12.4)	126 (6.0) 25 (6.9)
Religion	Other Islam	313 (12.1) 2128 (87.9)	19 (4.3) 163 (6.4)
Enabling/disabling factors			
Residence	Rural Urban	1252 (76.6) 1189 (23.4)	64 (5.2) 118 (9.1)
Health care visit (past 12 months)	No Yes	1037 (44.7) 1404 (55.3)	49 (4.4) 133 (7.5)
Education	No schooling <Primary Primary ≥Secondary	760 (36.9) 402 (16.0) 838 (33.1) 428 (13.9)	34 (3.7) 29 (5.0) 56 (6.0) 61 (13.9)
Current smokeless tobacco use	No Yes	1616 (67.6) 825 (32.4)	121 (5.6) 61 (7.2)
Fruit and vegetable intake (<5 servings/day)	No Yes	312 (10.4) 2086 (89.6)	26 (8.3) 155 (5.9)
Low physical activity	No Yes	2089 (88.4) 331 (11.6)	149 (6.1) 33 (7.1)
Need factors			
Central obesity	No Yes	1122 (50.9) 1263 (49.1)	51 (4.5) 129 (8.0)
Hypertension	No Yes	1700 (70.2) 735 (29.8)	116 (5.7) 66 (7.2)
Diabetes	No Yes	1959 (90.8) 209 (9.2)	135 (5.6) 27 (11.0)
Heart attack or stroke	No Yes	2153 (87.0) 288 (13.0)	140 (5.7) 42 (8.8)
Dyslipidaemia	No Yes	666 (32.7) 1494 (67.3)	37 (5.1) 124 (6.6)

Our findings

The sample included 2,441 women 30-49 years old. The majority (94.8%) of the participants were married, not employed (87.6%), were Muslim (87.9%) and lived in rural areas (76.6%). Almost two in five women (36.9%) had no formal education, 32.4% were current smokers of tobacco, 89.6% consumed inadequate fruit and vegetables and 11.6% engaged in low physical activity. Almost half of the women (49.1%) had central obesity, 29.8% had hypertension, 9.2% diabetes, 13.0% had a history of heart attack or stroke and 67.3% had dyslipidaemia. Only a low proportion of the women (6.1%) reported that they had ever undergone CCS (see Table 1).

Among those women who ever had CCS, 46.1% had CCS in the past two years. The main reasons for the last CCS were "experiencing pain or other symptoms" (43.6%) and recommended by a health care provider (37.6%). The location of the last CCS was the government hospital (42.3%) and the private hospital (41.2%), and the result of the last CCS was normal (55.6%), abnormal (17.6%) and suspect cancer (9.3%) (see Table 2).

Table 2. Characteristics of cervical cancer screening among women aged 30-49 years who ever screened (N = 182)

Variable	**Sub-category**	**N (%)**
Last cervical cancer test	<1 year ago	42 (23.1)
	1-2 years ago	60 (33.0)
	3-5 years ago	39 (21.4)
	>5 years ago	41 (22.5)
Main reason for last cervical cancer test	Experiencing pain or other symptoms	79 (43.6)
	Recommendation of health care provider	68 (37.6)
	Part of routine check up	11 (6.1)
	Other	23 (14.7)
Location of last cervical cancer test	Government hospital	77 (42.3)
	Private hospital	75 (41.2)
	Private doctor chamber	21 (11.5)
	Other	9 (4.8)
Result of last cervical cancer test	Normal	103 (55.6)
	Abnormal	32 (17.6)
	Suspect cancer	17 (9.3)
	Did not get result	20 (11.0)
	Inconclusive	6 (3.3)
	Do not know	4 (4.2)

Associations with cervical cancer screening uptake

In adjusted logistic regression analysis, health care provider visit in the past 12 months (AOR: 1.78, 95% CI: 1.12-1.82), and having secondary or higher education (AOR: 3.24, 95% CI: 1.60, 6.56), were positively associated with ever having had CCS. In addition, in unadjusted analysis, urban residence, having diabetes and central obesity increased the odds of CCS (see Table 3).

Table 3. Associations with ever cervical cancer screening among women aged 30-49 years

Variable	Sub-category	UOR (95% CI)	AOR (95% CI)
Predisposing factors			
Marital status	Not married Married	1 (Reference) 1.06 (0.44-2.55)	---
Work status	Not employed Employed	1 (Reference) 1.16 (0.59-2.31)	---
Religion	Other Islam	1 (Reference) 1.52 (0.81-2.86)	---
Enabling/disabling factors			
Residence	Rural Urban	1 (Reference) 1.81 (1.15-2.84)**	1 (Reference) 1.19 (0.72-1.96))
Health care visit (past 12 months)	No Yes	1 (Reference) 1.77 (1.17-2.20)**	1 (Reference) 1.78 (1.12-1.82)*
Education	No schooling <Primary Primary ≥Secondary	1 (Reference) 1.37 (0.73-2.58) 0.68 (0.94-2.99) 4.25 (2.32-7.79)***	1 (Reference) 1.25 (0.64-2.42) 1.41 (0.75-2.66) 3.24 (1.60-6.56)***
Current smokeless tobacco use	No Yes	1 (Reference) 2.30 (0.84-2.01)	---
Fruit and vegetable intake (<5 servings/day)	No Yes	1 (Reference) 0.70 (0.37-1.30)	---
Low physical activity	No Yes	1 (Reference) 1.18 (0.65-2.16)	---
Need factors			
Central obesity	No Yes	1 (Reference) 1.84 (1.12-3.01)*	1 (Reference) 1.56 (0.90-2.72)
Hypertension	No Yes	1 (Reference) 1.28 (0.84-1.99)	---
Diabetes	No Yes	1 (Reference) 2.07 (1.03-4.17)*	1 (Reference) 1.63 (0.79-3.39)
Heart attack or stroke	No Yes	1 (Reference) 1.49 (0.95-2.67)	---
Dyslipidaemia	No Yes	1 (Reference) 1.32 (0.74-2.32)	---

UOR = Unadjusted odds ratio; AOR = Adjusted odds ratio; $*p < 0.05$, $**p < 0.01$, $***p < 0.001$.

Discussion

In this national STEPS survey among Bangladeshi women, the prevalence of ever CCS (6.1%) was lower than in a survey in seven districts in Bangladesh (8.3%) (5), in Dhaka, Bangladesh (26%) (4) and in 55 LMICs (44%) (6). The result that almost half of the participants (43.6%) reported 'experiencing pain or other symptoms' as the main reason for the last CCS, shows the importance of increasing early CCS. The results are short of the national target to expand access and availability of CCS services in Bangladesh to 100% of women 30-60 years of age (2). Furthermore, the implementation and scale up of organized CCS through improved health service delivery and public awareness campaigns for the control of CC in Bangladesh are planned (2).

Consistent with some previous research (17-19), this study showed that a higher socioeconomic status (higher education) and urban residence increased the odds for CCS uptake. Higher education women may have better knowledge of CC health risks, which encourages them to seek CCS (17). Women residing in urban areas may have better access to CCS health care services than women who live in rural areas.

Unlike in a previous review (20), this study found in univariable analysis a positive (not negative) association between having obesity, diabetes and CCS, and no association between other chronic conditions, such as hypertension and dyslipidaemia. Women with excess weight may more likely utilize health services, which may increase the chances of CCS (21). Unlike previous research (19, 22), we did not find an association between other positive lifestyle behaviours and CCS.

Study limitations include that data on CCS and some other variables were assessed by self-report, and the cross-sectional study design. Future studies should include questions about the knowledge and attitudes about cancer and CCS.

Conclusion

The study showed that in this national survey only one in sixteen women (30-49 years) ever had CCS in Bangladesh. Several factors associated with CSS, including health care provider visit and having central obesity, that can be included in targeted interventions.

Acknowledgments

This paper uses data from the 2018 Bangladesh STEPS survey, implemented by the National Institute of Preventive and Social Medicine with the support of the World Health Organization.

References

[1] World Health Organization (WHO) Cervical cancer, 2020. URL: https://www.who.int/cancer/prevention/diagnosis-screening/cervical-cancer/en/.

[2] Government of the People's Republic of Bangladesh. National strategy for cervical cancer prevention and control, Bangladesh (2017-2022), 2017. URL: https://www.who.int/docs/default-source/searo/bangladesh/pdf-reports/cervical-cancer-strategy-english-book250118.pdf?sfvrsn=d00fcf51_2#:~:text=In%20 Bangladesh%2C%20Visual%20Inspection%20by,colposcopy%20test%20and%20treated%20accordingly.

[3] Hoque MR, Haque E, Karim MR. Cervical cancer in low-income countries: A Bangladeshi perspective. Int J Gynaecol Obstet 2021;152(1):19-25. doi: 10.1002/ijgo.13400.

[4] Qayum MO, Billah MM, Akhter R, Flora MS. Women's knowledge, attitude and practice on cervical cancer and its screening in Dhaka, Bangladesh. Asian Pac J Cancer Prev 2021;22(10):3327-35. doi: 10.31557/APJCP.2021.22.10.3327.

[5] Islam RM, Bell RJ, Billah B, Hossain MB, Davis SR. Lack of understanding of cervical cancer and screening is the leading barrier to screening uptake in women at midlife in Bangladesh: Population-based cross-sectional survey. Oncologist 2015;20(12):1386-92. doi: 10.1634/theoncologist.2015-0235.

[6] Lemp JM, De Neve JW, Bussmann H, Chen S, Manne-Goehler J, Theilmann M, et al. Lifetime prevalence of cervical cancer screening in 55 low- and middle-income cuntries. JAMA 2020;324(15):1532-42. doi: 10.1001/jama.2020.16244.

[7] Pengpid S, Peltzer K. Prevalence and risk factors for cervical and breast cancer screening among women in the general population in Indonesia. Gend Behav 2018;16(3):11994-003.

[8] Phaswana-Mafuya N, Peltzer K. Breast and cervical cancer screening prevalence and associated factors among women in the South African general population. Asian Pac J Cancer Prev 2018;19(6):1465-70. doi: 10.22034/APJCP.2018.19.6.1465.

[9] World Health Organization (WHO). STEPwise approach to surveillance (STEPS), 2018. URL: https://www.who.int/ncds/surveillance/steps/en/.

[10] World Health Organization. Country Office for Bangladesh. National STEPS survey for non-communicable diseases risk factors in Bangladesh, 2018. World Health Organization. Country Office for Bangladesh. URL: https://apps.who.int/iris/handle/10665/332886.

[11] Armstrong T, Bull F. Development of the World Health Organization Global Physical Activity Questionnaire (GPAQ). J Public Health 2006;14:66–70.

[12] Harvard School of Public Health. Abdominal obesity measurement guidelines for different ethnic groups, 2020. URL: https://www.hsph.harvard.edu/obesity-prevention-source/waist-circumference-guidelines-for-different-ethnic-groups/.

[13] Chobanian AV, Bakris GL, Black HR, Cushman WC, Green LA, Izzo JL et al. Seventh report of the Joint National Committee of Prevention, Detection, Evaluation, and Treatment of High Blood Pressure. Hypertension 2003;42(6):1206–52. http://dx.doi.org/10.1161/01.HYP.0000107251.49515.c2.

[14] World Health Organization (WHO) WHO STEPS Surveillance Manual. URL: https://www.who.int/ncds/surveillance/steps/STEPS_Manual.pdf.

[15] Expert Panel on Detection, Evaluation, and Treatment of High Blood Cholesterol in Adults. Executive Summary of the Third Report of the National Cholesterol Education Program (NCEP) Expert Panel on Detection, Evaluation, And Treatment of High Blood Cholesterol In Adults (Adult Treatment Panel III). JAMA 2001;285(19):2486-97. doi: 10.1001/jama.285.19.2486.

[16] World Health Organization. WHO guidelines for screening and treatment of precancerous lesions for cervical cancer prevention, 2019. URL: https://apps.who.int/ iris/bitstream/handle/10665/94830/ 9789241548694_eng.pdf.

[17] Ampofo AG, Adumatta AD, Owusu E, Awuviry-Newton K. A cross-sectional study of barriers to cervical cancer screening uptake in Ghana: An application of the health belief model. PLoS One 2020;15(4):e0231459. doi: 10.1371/journal.pone.0231459.

[18] Islam RM, Billah B, Hossain MN, Oldroyd J. Barriers to cervical cancer and breast cancer screening uptake in low-income and middle-income countries: A systematic review. Asian Pac J Cancer Prev 2017;18(7):1751-63. doi: 10.22034/APJCP.2017.18.7.1751.

[19] Sözmen K, Unal B, Sakarya S, Dinc G, Yardim N, Keskinkilic B, et al. Determinants of breast and cervical cancer screening uptake among women in Turkey. Asia Pac J Public Health 2016;28(6):528-38. doi: 10.1177/1010539516654541.

[20] Maruthur NM, Bolen SD, Brancati FL, Clark JM. The association of obesity and cervical cancer screening: a systematic review and meta-analysis. Obesity (Silver Spring) 2009;17(2):375-81. doi: 10.1038/oby.2008.480.

[21] Heflin MT, Oddone EZ, Pieper CF, Burchett BM, Cohen HJ. The effect of comorbid illness on receipt of cancer screening by older people. J Am Geriatr Soc 2002;50(10):1651-8. doi: 10.1046/j.1532-5415.2002.50456.x.

[22] Theme Filha MM, Leal MD, Oliveira EF, Esteves-Pereira AP, Gama SG. Regional and social inequalities in the performance of Pap test and screening mammography and their correlation with lifestyle: Brazilian national health survey, 2013. Int J Equity Health 2016;15(1):136. doi: 10.1186/s12939-016-0430-9.

Chapter 3

Perceived oral health status among adults in Mongolia: Prevalence and correlates of a national survey in 2019

Karl Peltzer*, **PhD**

Department of Psychology, University of the Free State, Bloemfontein, South Africa
Department of Psychology, College of Medical and Health Science, Asia University, Taichung, Taiwan

Abstract

The purpose of this analysis was to evaluate self-rated oral health (SROH) in a national community survey among adults in Mongolia. The study analysed national data from the Mongolian cross-sectional STEPS survey in 2019 (N = 6,654, 15-69 years). The assessment included physical measures, biochemistry tests and SROH, oral conditions, oral health behaviour, and general health behaviour and status. The results showed that the prevalence of poor SROH was 11.3%, 10.3 among women and 12.3% among men. In multivariable logistic regression analysis, a lower number of teeth (AOR: 5.58, 95% CI: 4.29-7.27), pain in the teeth, gum or mouth (AOR: 2.03, 95% CI: 1.55-2.66), current smoking tobacco (AOR: 1.57, 95% CI: 1.20-2.05) and insufficient fruit/vegetable consumption (AOR: 1.47, 95% CI: 1.08-2.01) were positively associated with poor SROH. Higher education (≥12 years) (AOR: 0.76, 95% CI: 0.59-0.98), teeth cleaning (≥2 times/day) (AOR: 0.75, 95% CI: 0.59-0.96), and the use of fluoride tooth paste (AOR: 0.63, 95% CI: 0.46-0.87) were protective against poor SROH. In addition, in unadjusted analysis, older age, male sex, dentures, recent dental visit,

* ***Correspondence:*** Professor Karl Peltzer, Department of Psychology, University of the Free State, PO Box 339 (40), Bloemfontein 9300, South Africa. Email: kfpeltzer@gmail.com.

In: Non-Communicable Diseases
Editor: Joav Merrick
ISBN: 979-8-89113-514-7

heavy episodic drinking, overweight/obesity, hypertension, diabetes, and heart attack or stroke were positively associated with poor SROH. More than one in ten adults in Mongolia had poor SROH and several associated factors were identified that can guide oral health promotion strategies in Mongolia.

Keywords: health status, self-rated oral health, health behaviour, Mongolia

Introduction

Oral diseases are a major public health concern, including in lower resourced countries (1). Worldwide, more than 2.2 billion people have dental caries and almost 10% have severe periodontal diseases (1). Other oral health conditions include oral cancers, cleft lip and palate, oro-dental trauma, noma, and oral manifestations of HIV (1). Poor oral health status negatively affects general health and well-being (2). Cosumer-oriented health care needs tp take the biopsychosocial dimension of oral health into account, including self-rated oral health (SROH) (2). Understanding the concept of SROH may assist in improving dental care provision (2), and has been shown to correlate with examined oral health status (3). Yet, we could find a study on SROH in Mongolia, a lower middle-income country in East Asia.

In the Mongolian "National Survey on Oral Health Status of Children and Adults" in 2016, the rate of dental morbidity was high, including 97.2% dental caries among urban and 98.5% among rural 35-44-year-olds, and the prevalence of gingivitis was 36.9% among urban and 35.5% among rural 35-44-year-olds (4). In national STEPS surveys, for example in Kenya, the prevalence of poor SROH was 13.7% (5), in Ecuador 9.7% (6), and in Sudan 8.0% (7). In local surveys in Asian countries, for example in rural Southern India, 15.2% reported poor SROH (8), and among middle-aged adults in Myanmar, 13.6% reported poor SROH (9). As reviewed previously (5):

> "factors associated with poor SROH include sociodemographic factors (older age, female and low socioeconomic status), oral conditions (toothache, dental caries, sensitive teeth, bad breath, bleeding gums, and reduced number of teeth), general health status (overweight and obesity and diabetes), oral health risk behaviour (inadequate tooth brushing, low oral hygiene behaviours, dental attendance), and general health risk behaviours (problem drinking, tobacco use, poor diets, food avoidance and physical inactivity)."

The study aims to assess SROH among individuals 15 years and older in the 2019 Mongolia STEPS survey.

Methods

Secondary data from the STEPS cross-sectional and nationally representative survey in Mongolia in 2019 were analysed (10). The overall study response rate was 98.1%; further study details can be accessed elsewhere (11).

Following the STEPS survey procedures, "Socio-demographic and behavioural information was collected in Step 1. Physical measurements such as height, weight, and blood pressure were collected in Step 2. Biochemical measurements were collected to assess blood glucose and cholesterol levels in Step 3 (12). A multi-stage stratified sampling process was carried out to randomly select participants from the target population (15-69 years). One individual within the age range of the survey (15-69 years) was selected per household (11). Ethics approval was provided by the Ministry of Health Medical Ethical Committee, Mongolia and written informed consent was obtained from all participants (11).

Study measures

SROH was sourced from the item, "How would you describe the state of your teeth?" (11). Poor SROH was defined as "having poor or very poor status of teeth, and good oral health as having average, good, very good or excellent status of teeth." (5-7).

Oral health-related behaviours were sourced from four items: 1) "How often do you clean your teeth?" ("1 = never to 7 twice or more a day"); 2) "Do you use toothpaste?"(Yes or No); 3) Do yo use tooth paste with fluoride?" (Yes, No, Do not know), and 4) "How long has it been since you last saw a dentist?" ("1 = less than 6 months to 6 = never received dental care") (11).

Oral conditions: "tooth loss defined as having 0-19 teeth (versus having 20 or more teeth)", dentures, "Do you have any removable dentures?" ("Yes, No"), and physical symptoms: "During the past 12 months, did your teeth, gums or mouth cause any pain, swelling, bleeding or discomfort?" ("Yes/No") (11).

Hypertension (BP) was defined as "systolic BP ≥140 mm Hg and/or diastolic BP ≥90 mm Hg or currently on antihypertensive medication" (mean of the last two of three measurements) (12, 13), and general overweight/ obesity (measured body mass index: "overweight 23.0-24.9 kg/m^2, obesity ≥25.0 kg/m^2" (14). Diabetes was defined as "fasting plasma glucose levels ≥7.0 mmol/L, and/or currently taking insulin or oral hypoglycemic drugs" (12).

Health risk behaviours included current smoking, daily fruit and vegetable intake, current heavy episodic drinking ("six or more standard drinks on a single occasion of drinking"), sedentary behaviour (≥8 hours/day) and levels of physical activity based on the "Global Physical Activity Questionnaire" (15). Sociodemographic data consisted of education, sex, age, ethnic group and residence status (11). A history of cardiovascular disease (CVD) included self-reported "Have you ever had a heart attack or chest pain from heart disease (angina) or a stroke (cerebrovascular accident or incident)? (Yes, No)" (11).

Statistical analysis

STATA software version 13.0 software (Stata Corporation, College Station, TX, USA) was used for statistical analyses, taking the multi-stage sampling and weighting of the data into account. Frequencies and percentages were calculated to describe the data. Logistic regression was applied to model factors (social, oral conditions, oral health behaviour, health risk behaviour and health status indicators) associated with poor SROH. $p < 0.05$ was considered significant. Variables significant in univariable analysis were subsequently included in the multivariable model.

Results

The sample included 6,654 people aged 15-69 years, 55.4% were women, 64.8% lived in urban areas, and 46.2% had 12 or more years of education. In terms of oral conditions, 28.6% had removable dentures, 29.8% had < 20 natural teeth, and 33.0% had dental pain (past year). More than half of the participants (55.9%) cleaned their teeth ≥2 times/day, 76.4% used fluoride toothpaste, and 35.2% had visited a dentist in the past year. General health risk behaviour included 24.6% current tobacco smoking, 21.4% heavy episodic drinking, 80.6% insufficient fruit/vegetable consumption, and 29.9% had low physical activity. More than two in three participants (71.9%) had overweight or obesity, 29.2% hypertension, 9.6% diabetes, and 15.8% had a history of heart attack or stroke. The prevalence of poor SROH was 11.3%, 10.3 among women, and 12.3% among men (see Table 1).

Associations with poor SROH

In multivariable logistic regression analysis, a lower number of teeth (AOR: 5.58, 95% CI: 4.29-7.27), pain in the teeth, gum or mouth (AOR: 2.03, 95% CI: 1.55-2.66), current smoking tobacco (AOR: 1.57, 95% CI: 1.20-2.05), and inadequate fruit/vegetable consumption (AOR: 1.47, 95% CI: 1.08-2.01) were positively associated with poor SROH. Higher education (≥12 years) (AOR: 0.76, 95% CI: 0.59-0.98), teeth cleaning (≥2 times/day) (AOR: 0.75, 95% CI: 0.59-0.96), and the use of fluoride tooth paste (AOR: 0.63, 95% CI: 0.46-0.87) were protective against poor SROH. Additionally, in the unadjusted analysis, older age, male sex, dentures, recent dental visit, heavy episodic drinking, overweight/obesity, hypertension, diabetes, and heart attack or stroke were positively associated with poor SROH (see Table 2).

Discussion

The aim of the study was to evaluate poor SROH and associated factors in a sample of a national general adult population in Mongolia. We found a prevalence of poor SROH (11.3%), which appears lower than in some other studies in Asia, eg, rural India (15.2%) (8) and Myanmar (13.6%) (9), but higher than, for example, in Sudan (8.0%) (7), Brazil (5.9%) (16), and Ecuador (9.7%) (6). The high prevalence of poor SROH may mirror a high prevalence of dental morbidity in Mongolia, as previously found (4).

Consistent with some previous research (7, 17-19), we found lower education and older age in unadjusted analysis were associated with poor SROH. Lower general education may also impact on lower oral health behaviour increasing poor SROH (6). Some previous studies found an association between female sex (7, 17), ethnicity (6), urban residence (7) and poor SROH, while in adjusted analysis we did not find significant differences in the prevalence of poor SROH in terms of sex, residence and ethnicity.

Consistent with previous research (20-22), the survey showed that oral conditions (tooth loss and pain in the teeth, gums, or mouth), increased the odds of poor SROH. Of concern is that the prevalence of oral conditions was high, e.g., <20 teeth 29.9%, compared to Kenya (2.2%) (5), and Sudan (10.8%) (7), removable dentures 28.6%, compared to Kenya (4.6%) (5), and Sudan (1.3%) (7), past 12-month pain in teeth, gums or mouth 33.0%, compared to Kenya (31.6%) (5), and Sudan (23.1%) (7). The higher prevalence of oral conditions in this study may in part explain the high prevalence of poor SROH.

Furthermore, several oral health behaviours (teeth cleaning ≥2 times/day, and using tooth paste with fluoride) decreased the odds of poor SROH, which is consistent with previous research (21, 23, 24). However, there is a concern that only 55.9% of the participants cleened their teeth regularly, 76.4% used toothpaste with fluoride, and 35.2% had a dental care visit in the past 12 months. In comparison, for example in Ecuador (6), 85.1% cleened their teeth ≥2 times/day, and 98.6% used toothpaste with fluoride. This could imply that special efforts should be made in Mongolia to promote oral health behaviours to improve oral health.

In terms of general health risk behaviours, we found, in agreement with previous research in terms of smoking tobacco (8, 25, 26) and poor diet (26, 27), that smoking tobacco and inadequate fruit and vegetable intake were positively associated with poor SROH. However, unlike some previous results (28, 29), heavy alcohol use and physical inactivity were not significantly associated with poor SROH. These results seem to partially confirm a clustering of oral and general health-risk behaviours (30).

Some previous research found an association between general health status [overweight/obesity (31, 32), diabetes (17), and heart attack or stroke (6)] and poor SROH, which we only found in unadjusted analysis for diabetes, overweight/obesity, stroke or heart attack and hypertension.

Study limitations include that oral health and some other variales were assessed by self-report, which may have led to biased responses, and due to the cross-sectional study design no causal inferences can be made. Future research may include objective and subjective oral health status assessments. The variable on household income had too many missing cases and was therefore excluded from the analysis. In addition, additional dietary questions, such as consumption of sugar sweetened beverages and sugar, were not included and should form part of future research.

Table 1. Sample and oral health characteristics, Mongolia STEPS survey, 2019

Variables	Subcategories	Sample	Self-rated poor oral health
		N (% unweighted)	% weighted
All		6654	11.3
Age group (in years)	15-29	1473 (22.1)	6.7
	30-44	2491 (37.4)	9.7
	45-69	2690 (40.4)	20.0
Sex	Female	3688 (55.4)	10.3
	Male	2966 (44.6)	12.3
Education (in years)	0-9	1868 (28.1)	16.3
	10-11	1712 (25.7)	12.9
	≥12	3074 (46.2)	8.0
Ethnicity	Other	1005 (15.2)	11.3
	Khalkh	5621 (84.8)	11.2
Household adult members	0-2	3680 (55.9)	10.6
	3 or more	2906 (44.1)	11.7
Residence	Rural	2339 (35.2)	11.3
	Urban	4315 (64.8)	11.2
Number of teeth	20 or more	4632 (70.2)	6.2
	0-19	1962 (29.8)	31.2
Dentures (removable)	Yes	1900 (28.6)	22.3
Pain in teeth/gum/mouth (past year)	Yes	2192 (33.0)	14.9
Teeth cleaning	≥twice/day	3717 (55.9)	8.5
Uses toothpaste	Yes	6459 (98.0)	11.0
Tooth paste with fluoride	No	705 (10.9)	15.0
	Do not know	822 (12.7)	14.3
	Yes	4932 (76.4)	9.8
Dentist consultation	Never	671 (10.1)	7.9
	>12 months ago	3638 (54.7)	10.9
	Past 12 months	2343 (35.2)	12.8
Current smoking tobacco	Yes	1638 (24.6)	16.2
Heavy episodic drinking	Yes	1397 (21.4)	14.3
Inadequate fruit and vegetable intake	Yes	5105 (80.6)	11.9
Physical activity	Low	1957 (29.9)	12.5
	Moderate	1226 (18.7)	13.3
	High	3356 (51.3)	10.0
Overweight/obesity	Yes	4630 (71.9)	12.3
Hypertension	Yes	1922 (29.2)	16.9
Diabetes	Yes	604 (9.6)	16.2
Stroke or heart attack	Yes	1051 (15.8)	14.6

Table 2. Simple and multivariable logistic regression with poor self-rated oral health status

Variables	Subcategories	COR (95% CI)	AOR (95% CI)
Age group (in years)	15-29	1 (Reference)	1 (Reference)
	30-44	1.50 (1.10, 2.04)*	1.05 (0.74, 1.47)
	45-69	3.49 (2.60, 4.69)***	0.91 (0.62, 1.32)
Sex	Female	1 (Reference)	1 (Reference)
	Male	1.22 (1.03, 1.44)*	1.06 (0.82, 1.36)
Education (in years)	0-9	1 (Reference)	1 (Reference)
	10-11	0.76 (0.61, 0.96)*	0.94 (0.72, 1.22)
	≥12	0.44 (0.36, 0.55)***	0.76 (0.59, 0.98)*
Ethnicity	Other	1 (Reference)	---
	Khalkh	0.99 (0.77, 1.28)	
Household adult members	0-2	1 (Reference)	---
	3 or more	1.13 (0.95, 1.34)	
Residence	Rural	1 (Reference)	---
	Urban	1.11 (0.89, 1.36)	
Number of teeth	20 or more	1 (Reference)	1 (Reference)
	0-19	6.85 (5.61, 8.38)***	5.58 (4.29, 7.27)***
Dentures (removable)	Yes	3.05 (2.53, 3.67)***	1.24 (0.96, 1.60)
Pain in teeth/gum/mouth (past year)	Yes	1.71 (1.39, 2.10)***	2.03 (1.55, 2.66)***
Teeth cleaning	≥twice/day	0.53 (0.43, 0.65)***	0.75 (0.59, 0.96)*
Tooth paste with fluoride	No	1 (Reference)	1 (Reference)
	Do not know	0.94 (0.67, 1.34)	0.79 (0.51, 1.21)
	Yes	0.61 (0.47, 0.80)***	0.63 (0.46, 0.87)**
Dentist consultation	Never	1 (Reference)	1 (Reference)
	>12 months ago	1.43 (1.00, 2.04)	1.30 (0.86, 1.98)
	Past 12 months	1.72 (1.20, 2.46)**	1.18 (0.76, 1.83)
Current smoking tobacco	Yes	1.79 (1.49, 2.17)***	1.57 (1.20, 2.05)***
Heavy episodic drinking	Yes	1.41 (1.14, 1.74)***	1.09 (0.83, 1.43)
Inadequate fruit and vegetable intake	Yes	1.41 (1.09, 1.83)**	1.47 (1.08, 2.01)*
Physical activity	Low	1 (Reference)	---
	Moderate	1.07 (0.84, 1.38)	
	High	0.78 (0.64, 0.95)	
Overweight/obesity	Yes	1.28 (1.02, 1.61)*	0.90 (0.69, 1.18)
Hypertension	Yes	1.89 (1.57, 2.29)***	1.01 (0.79, 1.28)
Diabetes	Yes	1.56 (1.16, 2.08)**	1.21 (0.84, 1.74)
Stroke or heart attack	Yes	1.42 (1.11, 1.82)**	1.19 (0.89, 1.61)

$*p < 0.05$, $**p < 0.01$, $***p < 0.001$; COR = Crude Odds Ratio; AOR = Adjusted Odds Ratio; CI = Confidence Interval.

Conclusion

More than one in ten adults in Mongolia had poor SROH and several associated factors were identified, including poor oral conditions (having <20 teeth, and pain in teeth, gums or mouth), poor oral health behaviour (<twice a day teeth cleaning and not using toothpaste with fluoride), general health risk behaviour (current smoking tobacco and inadequate fruit and vegetable intake), that can guide oral health promotion strategies in Mongolia.

Acknowledgments

"This paper uses data from the 2019 Mongolia STEPS survey, implemented by the Ministry of Health with the support of the World Health Organization."

References

[1] World Health Organization. Factsheet, Oral health, 2020. URL: https://www.who.int/news-room/fact-sheets/detail/oral-health.

[2] Petersen PE, Bourgeois D, Ogawa H, Estupinan-Day S, Ndiaye C. The global burden of oral diseases and risks to oral health. Bull World Health Organ 2005;83(9):661-9.

[3] Blizniuk A, Ueno M, Zaitsu T, Kawaguchi Y. Association between self-reported and clinical oral health status in Belarusian adults. J Investig Clin Dent 2017;8(2). doi: 10.1111/jicd.12206.

[4] Delgertsetseg J, Oyuntsetseg B, Munkh-Od S, Suvdanchimeg A, Amarsaikhan B. The results of national oral health survey, Mongolia. Cent Asian J Med Sci 2018;4:61–8.

[5] Pengpid S, Peltzer K. Self-rated oral health status and social and health determinants among community dwelling adults in Kenya. Afr Health Sci 2019;19(4):3146-53. doi: 10.4314/ahs.v19i4.37.

[6] Pengpid S, Peltzer K. Prevalence and associated factors of self-rated oral health among a national population-based sample of adults in Ecuador: Results of the 2018 STEPS survey. J Int Oral Health 2021;13:122-8. doi: 10.4103/jioh.jioh_313_20.

[7] Pengpid S, Peltzer K. Prevalence and associated factors of self-rated oral health among a national population-based sample of adults in Sudan: Results of the 2016 STEPS survey. Oral Health Prev Dent 2021;19(1):391-7. doi: 10.3290/j.ohpd.b1749751.

[8] Bhat M, Bhat S, Roberts-Thomson KF, Do LG. Self-rated oral health and associated factors among an adult population in rural India: An epidemiological study. Int J Environ Res Public Health 2021;18(12):6414. doi: 10.3390/ijerph18126414.

[9] Jayasvasti I, Htun KCSS, Peltzer K. Self-rated oral health status and social and health determinants among 35-65 year-old persons in one region In Myanmar: A cross-sectional study. Clin Cosmet Investig Dent 2019;11:339-48. doi: 10.2147/CCIDE.S227957.

[10] World Health Organization (WHO). STEPwise approach to surveillance (STEPS), 2020. URL: https://www.who.int/ncds/surveillance/steps/en/.

[11] National Centre for Public Health. Fourth national STEPS survey on prevalence of non-communicable disease and injury risk factors-2019, 2020. Ulaanbaatar: National Centre for Public Health. URL: https://extranet.who.int/ncdsmicrodata/index.php/catalog/836/related-materials.

[12] World Health Organization (WHO). WHO STEPS surveillance manual. URL: https://www.who.int/ncds/surveillance/steps/STEPS_Manual.pdf.

[13] Chobanian AV, Bakris GL, Black HR, Cushman WC, Green LA, Izzo JL et al. Seventh report of the Joint National Committee of Prevention, Detection, Evaluation, and Treatment of High Blood Pressure. Hypertension 2003;42(6):1206–52. http://dx.doi.org/10.1161/01.HYP.0000107251.49515.c2.

[14] Wen CP, David Cheng TY, Tsai SP, Chan HT, Hsu HL, et al. Are Asians at greater mortality risks for being overweight than Caucasians? Redefining obesity for Asians. Public Health Nutr 2009;12(4):497-506. doi: 10.1017/S1368980008002802.

[15] Armstrong T, Bull F. Development of the World Health Organization Global Physical Activity Questionnaire (GPAQ). J Public Health 2006;14:66–70.

[16] Sousa JL, Henriques A, Silva ZPD, Severo M, Silva S. Posição socioeconômica e autoavaliação da saúde bucal no Brasil: resultados da Pesquisa Nacional de Saúde [Socioeconomic position and self-rated oral health in Brazil: results of the Brazilian National Health Survey]. Cad Saude Publica 2019;35(6):e00099518. doi: 10.1590/0102-311X00099518. [Portuguese]

[17] Cheema S, Maisonneuve P, Al-Thani MH, et al. Oral health behavior and factors associated with poor oral status in Qatar: results from a national health survey. J Public Health Dent 2017;77(4):308-16. doi: 10.1111/jphd.12209.

[18] Olutola BG, Ayo-Yusuf OA. Socio-environmental factors associated with self-rated oral health in South Africa: a multilevel effects model. Int J Environ Res Public Health 2012;9(10):3465-83. doi: 10.3390/ijerph9103465.

[19] Vale EB, Mendes Ada C, Moreira Rda S. Self-perceived oral health among adults in Northeastern Brazil. Rev Saude Publica 2013;47(Suppl 3):98-108.

[20] Jones JA, Kressin NR, Spiro A 3rd, Randall CW, Miller DR, Hayes C, et al. Self-reported and clinical oral health in users of VA health care. J Gerontol A Biol Sci Med Sci 2001;56:M55-62.

[21] Arantes R, Frazão P. Subjective oral symptoms associated with self-rated oral health among Indigenous groups in Central-West Brazil. Commun Dent Oral Epidemiol 2018; 46:352-9. doi: 10.1111/cdoe.12375.

[22] Pattussi MP, Peres KG, Boing AF, Peres MA, da Costa JS. Self-rated oral health and associated factors in Brazilian elders. Commun Dent Oral Epidemiol 2010;38:348-59. doi: 10.1111/j.1600-0528.2010.00542.x.

[23] Afonso-Souza G, Nadanovsky P, Chor D, Faerstein E, Werneck GL, Lopes CS. Association between routine visits for dental checkup and self-perceived oral health in an adult population in Rio de Janeiro: the Pró-Saúde Study. Commun Dent Oral Epidemiol 2007;35:393-400.

[24] Andrade FB, Lebrão ML, Santos JL, Duarte YA, Teixeira DS. Factors related to poor self-perceived oral health among community-dwelling elderly individuals in São Paulo, Brazil. Cad Saude Publica 2012;28:1965-75.

[25] Olusile AO, Adeniyi AA, Orebanjo O. Self-rated oral health status, oral health service utilization, and oral hygiene practices among adult Nigerians. BMC Oral Health 2014;14:140. doi: 10.1186/1472-6831-14-140.

[26] Liu Y. The relationship between lifestyle and self-reported oral health among American adults. Int Dent J 2014;64:46-51. doi: 10.1111/idj.12061.

[27] Quandt SA, Chen H, Bell RA, Savoca MR, Anderson AM, Leng X, et al. Food avoidance and food modification practices of older rural adults: association with oral health status and implications for service provision. Gerontologist 2010;50(1):100-11. doi: 10.1093/geront/gnp096.

[28] Mejia G, Armfield JM, Jamieson LM. Self-rated oral health and oral health-related factors: the role of social inequality. Aust Dent J 2014;59:226-33. doi: 10.1111/adj.12173.

[29] Novak D, Štefan L, Emeljanovas A, Mieziene B, Milanović I, Janić SR, et al. Factors associated with good self-rated health in European adolescents: A population-based cross-sectional study. Int J Public Health 2017;62:971-9. doi: 10.1007/s00038-017-1015-0.

[30] Kobal G, Heynekamp J, Langston TB, Reeh P, Mishra MK, Flora JW. Inhibition of sensory irritation during consumption of non-smokeable tobacco products, 2018. URL: https://patents.google.com/patent/US10117453B2/en.

[31] Peltzer K, Pengpid S. Dental health status and oral health behavior among university students from five ASEAN countries. Nagoya J Med Sci 2017;79:123-33. doi: 10.18999/nagjms.79.2.123.

[32] Ekbäck G, Näslund I, Montgomery SM, Ordell S. Self-perceived oral health and obesity among 65 years old in two Swedish counties. Swed Dent J 2010;34:207-15.

Submitted: August 28, 2022. *Revised:* September 12, 2022. *Accepted:* September 17, 2022.

Chapter 4

Prevalence and correlates of intention to quit smoking among Jordanians and Syrians in Jordan: Results of a national STEPS survey in 2019

Supa Pengpid*, DrPH

Department of Health Education and Behavioral Sciences, Faculty of Public Health, Mahidol University, Bangkok, Thailand
Department of Public Health, Sefako Makgatho Health Sciences University, Pretoria, South Africa

Abstract

In this chapter we aimed to estimate the prevalence and associated factors of intention to quit smoking among adults in Jordan in 2019. National data was analysed from 5,713 adults (50.9% Jordanians and 49.1% Syrians) aged 18 to 69 years (mean 36.7) who participated in the cross-sectional "2019 Jordan STEPS survey." The results indicate that 31.5% of the participants intend to quit smoking, 30.8% among Jordanians, and 39.8% among Syrians. In adjusted logistic regression analysis, compared to Syrian participants, Jordanian participants were less likely to have the intention to quit smoking (AOR: 0.67, 95% CI: 0.49-0.92). Furthermore, past year smoking quit attempt (AOR: 2.51, 95% CI: 1.70-3.71) and having noticed health warnings on cigarette smoking in the newspaper (AOR: 1.89, 95% CI: 1.12-3.20) were positively associated with the intention to quit smoking. In addition, in unadjusted analysis, past year medical advice to stop smoking, TV, radio and internet and social media

* ***Correspondence:*** Professor Supa Pengpid, Department of Health Education and Behavioral Sciences, Faculty of Public Health, Mahidol University, 420/1 Ratchawithi Road, Ratchathewi, Bangkok 10400, Thailand. Email: supaprom@yahoo.com.

In: Non-Communicable Diseases
Editor: Joav Merrick
ISBN: 979-8-89113-514-7

exposure about the "dangers of smoking cigarettes or that encourages quitting" were associated with intention to quit smoking. About one in three adults in Jordan intend to quit smoking, and several associated factors were identified that can assist in planning interventions.

Introduction

Tobacco causes the death of eight million persons per year (1). The majority of the world's smokers (80%) live in lower resourced countries (1). Despite the harm of tobacco use, there is a high prevalence of tobacco smoking in Jordan. In a cross-sectional in five regional governorates of Jordan (18–79 years), current smoking was among men 59.1% and among women 23.3% (2). In a Global Adult Tobacco Survey (GATS) in Jordan in 2011, 42.2% of people aged 15 years and over smoked tobacco (3). In a local survey among adults in Amman, Jordan, in 2009-2010, 42% of current smokers considered quitting in the next 30 days (4). In order for smokers to minimize or avoid the harmful effects of smoking is to quit smoking (5). An important step for smokers to stop smoking is to have intentions to quit smoking (6). We lack recent and national data on intentions to quit smoking in Jordan.

"Jordan adopted the national tobacco control strategy for 2017-2019, which is based on the implementation of the WHO's MPOWER strategy, a comprehensive set of tobacco control measures" and is implemented to some extent (7). For example, the law mandates that "health warnings appear on tobacco packages (in case of cigarettes 40% of display areas), conduct of anti-tobacco mass media campaigns aired on television and/or radio, a toll-free telephone quit line/help line with a live person available to discuss cessation with callers, and in a few clinics smoking cessation services are available in Jordan" (8).

In the Global Adult Tobacco Surveys (GATS) in India in 2016-2017, 52.2% of current tobacco users were willing to quit tobacco use (9), which was 50.9% in an earlier survey in GATS 2009-2010 (10). In Kazakhstan the pevalence of intention to quit smoking was 75.9% among smokers (11), and in Malaysia, 85.2% of smokers intended to quit smoking (12). Among older adult smokers in South Korea 26.3% had the intention to quit smoking (13), and among adult smokers in Lebanon the intention to quit smoking was 24% (14).

Factors associated with intention to quit smoking include sociodemographic factors, tobacco related factors and use of other substances.

Sociodemographic factors include younger age groups (9), male sex (15), lower education (15), and higher education (9, 12). Tobacco related factors include a history of attempts to quit smoking (4, 6), receipt of health care advice to quit (9, 12), the use of one type of tobacco (9), the heaviness of smoking (4) and the exposure to anti-tobacco media messages (4, 9, 15). Other substance use factors associated include, for example, that heavy alcohol use was inversely associated with intention to quit smoking in Nepal (6). The study aimed to estimate the prevalence and associated factors of intention to quit smoking among adults in Jordan in 2019.

Our study

National cross-sectional data from the 2019 Jordan STEPS survey (16) were analysed; the study response rate was 95% (17). A multi-stage stratified sampling process was carried out to randomly select participants from the target population of adult Jordanians and Syrians. One individual within the age range of the survey (18-69 years) was selected per household. Ethics approval was provided by the Ethics Committee of the Jordan Ministry of Health for Scientific Research, and written informed consent was obtained from all participants" (16, 17).

Measures

Current smoking status was assessed with two questions, 1) "Do you currently smoke any tobacco products, such as cigarettes, cigars, pipes, or shisha?" (Yes/No) and 2) "Do you currently smoke tobacco products daily?" (Yes/No) (17).

"During the past 12 months, have you tried to stop smoking?" (Yes/No)

"During any visit to a doctor or other health worker in the past 12 months, were you advised to quit smoking tobacco?" (Yes/no/no visit) (coded 1 = yes, 0 = no/no visit)

"During the past 30 days, have you noticed information about the dangers of smoking cigarettes or that encourages quitting through the following media?" Newspapers, Television, Radio, Internet and Social Media (Yes/no/do not know) (coded 1 = yes, 0 = no/do not know) (17).

Current smokers were asked "During the past 30 days, did you notice any health warnings on cigarette packages?" (Yes/no/do not know) (coded 1 = yes, 0 = no/do not know), and health warnings aware participants were asked "During the past 30 days, have warning labels on cigarette packages led you to think about quitting?" (Yes/no/do not know) (coded 1 = yes, 0 = no/do not know) (17).

Further, current smokeless tobacco use was assessed with the question "Do you currently use any smokeless tobacco products such as snuff, chewing tobacco?" (Yes/No). History of alcohol use was measured with the item, "Have you ever consumed any alcohol such as beer, wine, spirits?" (Yes/No) (17).

Socioeconomic information consisted of education, sex, age, region, nationality, residence and "monthly household income in Jordanian Dinar (JD) (1st June 2019: $1 *USD* = JD 0.709)" (17).

All statistical analyses were conducted with "STATA software version 14.0 (Stata Corporation, College Station, TX, USA)." "Analysis weights were calculated by taking the inverse of the probability of selection of each participant. These weights were adjusted for differences in the age-sex composition of the sample population compared to the target population." (17). Descriptive statistics are used to describe the intention to quit smoking. Logistic regressions were applied to estimate predictors of intention to quit among health warning aware. P-values < 0.05 were considered significant.

Our findings

The sample included 5,713 adults (50.9% Jordanians and 49.1% Syrians) aged 18 to 69 years (mean 36.7, SD = 14.0). Majority were females (61.4%), living in the central region (56.5%) and resided in urban areas (81.3%). In total, 41.0% of the participants were current smokers. More details are provided in Table 1.

Distribution of intention to quit smoking

In all, 31.5% intented to quit smoking, 30.8% among Jordanians and 39.8% smong Syrians, and 41.9% with those who had tempted to quit smoking in the past year (see Table 2).

Table 1. Sample characteristics, Jordan 2019

Variable	Subcategory	Jordanian N (%[a])	Syrian N (%[a])	All N (%[a])
Total		**2910 (50.9)**	**2803 (49.1)**	**5713**
Age (years)	18-29	724 (24.9)	878 (31.3)	1602 (28.0)
	30-44	939 (32.3)	1207 (43.1)	2146 (37.6)
	45-59	819 (28.1)	520 (18.6)	1339 (23.4)
	60-69	428 (14.7)	198 (7.1)	626 (11.0)
Gender	Female	1712 (58.8)	1798 (64.1)	3510 (61.4)
	Male	1198 (41.2)	1005 (35.9_	2203 (38.6)
Education (in years)	0-6	453 (15.6)	1122 (40.0)	1575 (27.6)
	7-11	863 (29.7)	1091 (38.9)	1954 (34.2)
	≥12	1594 (54.8)	590 (21.0)	2184 (38.2)
Monthly household income (in Jordanian Dinar)	< 200	346 (12.8)	928 (36.6)	1274 (24.3)
	200-349	931 (34.4)	1199 (47.2)	2130 (40.6)
	≥350	1428 (52.8)	411 (16.2)	1839 (35.1)
Residence	Rural	567 (19.5)	501 (17.9)	2068 (18.7)
	Urban	2343 (80.5)	2302 (82.1)	4645 (81.3)
Region	Center	1708 (58.7)	1521 (54.3)	3229 (56.5)
	North	904 (31.1)	1282 (45.7)	2186 (38.3)
	South	298 (10.2)	---	298 (5.2)
Current smokers	No	1881 (48.0[b])	2031 (67.8[b])	3912 (59.0[b])
	Yes	1029 (42.0[b])	772 (32.[b])	1801 (41.0[b])

[a]Unweighted, [b]weighted.

Associations with intentions to quit smoking among health warning aware

In adjusted logistic regression analysis, compared to Syrian participants, Jordanian participants were less likely to have the intention to quit smoking (AOR: 0.67, 95% CI: 0.49-0.92). Furthermore, past year smoking quit attempt (AOR: 2.51, 95% CI: 1.70-3.71) and noticed health warnings on cigarette smoking in the newspaper (AOR: 1.89, 95% CI: 1.12-3.20) were positively associated with the intention to quit smoking. In addition, in unadjusted analysis, past year medical advice to stop smoking, TV, radio and internet and social media exposure about the "dangers of smoking cigarettes or that encourages quitting" were associated with intention to quit smoking (see Table 3).

Table 2. Distribution of intention to quit smoking among health warning aware

Variable	Subcategory	Intention to quit among health warning aware N (%)
Total		1368 (31.5)
Age (years)	18-29 (42.9%)	114 (30.0)
	30-44 (35.5%)	209 (32.9)
	45-59 (15.8%)	120 (30.5)
	60-69 (5.8%)	37 (37.1)
Gender	Female (19.9%)	106 (28.6)
	Male (80.1%)	374 (32.3)
Education (in years)	0-6 (12.5%)	121 (27.8)
	7-11 (39.4%)	203 (32.0)
	≥12 (48.1%)	156 (32.1)
Monthly household income (in Jordanian Dinar)	< 200 (9.8%)	96 (35.0)
	200-349 (32.8%)	181 (30.0)
	≥350 (57.4%)	166 (30.1)
Nationality	Syrian (8.4%)	227 (39.8)
	Jordanian (91.6%)	253 (30.8)
Residence	Rural (16.1%)	77 (27.3)
	Urban (83.9%)	403 (32.4)
Region	Center (60.8%)	276 (31.6)
	North (28.6%)	181 (32.6)
	South (10.6%)	23 (28.6)
Smoking frequency	< daily (15.6%)	83 (39.7)
	Daily (84.4%)	397 (30.2)
Past year smoking quit attempt	No (55.1%)	161 (22.2)
	Yes (44.9%)	319 (41.9)
Past year medical advice to stop smoking	No (71.7%)	230 (28.3)
	Yes (28.3%)	181 (37.8)
Current smokeless tobacco use	No (99.5%)	479 (31.7)
	Yes (0.5%	1 (9.7)
Ever alcohol use	No (88.4%)	425 (31.0)
	Yes (11.6%)	55 (35.7)
Notice health warning in newspaper	No (84.0%)	385 (28.7)
	Yes (16.0%)	95 (45.2)
Notice health warning in TV	No (63.0%)	240 (27.0)
	Yes (37.0%)	240 (38.7)
Notice health warning in radio	No (84.1%)	404 (30.0)
	Yes (15.9%)	76 (40.3)
Notice health warning in internet and social media	No (54.6%)	222 (26.3)
	Yes (45.4%)	258 (37.4)

Table 3. Associations with intention to quit among health warnings aware

Variable	Subcategory	Crude Odds Ratio (95% CI)	Adjusted Odds Ratio (95% CI)
Age (years)	18-29	1 (Reference)	---
	30-44	1.14 (0.76-1.72)	
	45-59	1.03 (0.66-1.59)	
	60-69	1.38 (0.74-2.57)	
Gender	Female	1 (Reference)	---
	Male	1.19 (0.80-1.76)	
Education (in years)	0-6	1 (Reference)	---
	7-11	1.22 (0.78-1.94)	
	≥12	1.23 (0.77-1.97)	
Monthly household income (in Jordanian Dinar)	< 200	1 (Reference)	---
	200-349	0.80 (0.47-1.35)	
	≥350	0.80 (0.47-1.34)	
Nationality	Syrian	1 (Reference)	1 (Reference)
	Jordanian	0.67 (0.51-0.90)**	0.67 (0.49-0.92)*
Residence	Rural	1 (Reference)	---
	Urban	1.28 (0.79-2.07)	
Region	Center	1 (Reference)	---
	North	1.05 (0.75-1.47)	
	South	0.87 (0.43-1.75)	
Smoking frequency	< daily	1 (Reference)	---
	Daily	0.66 (0.43-1.01)	
Current smokeless tobacco use	No	1 (Reference)	---
	Yes	0.23 (0.03-2.12)	
Ever alcohol use	No	1 (Reference)	---
	Yes	1.24 (0.78-1.98)	

Table 3. (Continued)

Variable	Subcategory	Crude Odds Ratio (95% CI)	Adjusted Odds Ratio (95% CI)
Past year smoking quit attempt	No	1 (Reference)	1 (Reference)
	Yes	2.53 (1.82-3.53)***	2.51 (1.70-3.71)***
Past year medical advice to stop smoking	No	1 (Reference)	1 (Reference)
	Yes	1.54 (1.06-2.24)*	1.36 (0.93-1.97)
Notice health warning in newspaper	No	1 (Reference)	1 (Reference)
	Yes	2.05 (1.25-3.12)***	1.89 (1.12-3.20)*
Notice health warning in TV	No	1 (Reference)	1 (Reference)
	Yes	1.71 (1.22-2.40)**	1.25 (0.81-1.92)
Notice health warning in radio	No	1 (Reference)	1 (Reference)
	Yes	1.57 (1.02-2.42)*	1.02 (0.61-1.68)
Notice health warning in internet and social media	No	1 (Reference)	1 (Reference)
	Yes	1.68 (1.21-2.32)**	1.32 (0.88-2.00)

CI = Confidence Interval; ***$p < 0.001$;**$p < 0.01$; *$p < 0.05$.

Discussion

The study found in a national sample of Jordanians and Syrians (18-69 years) in 2019 in Jordan that the prevalence of current smoking (41.0%) was similar to a study in five regional governorates of Jordan (59.1% among men and 23.3% among women) (6), and the Jordan Global Adult Tobacco Survey (GATS) in 2011 (42.2%) (3). This means that despite Jordan's adoption of the national tobacco control strategy with a comprehensive set of tobacco control measures (7), no reduction in the prevalence of tobacco smoking was achieved over the past 10 years.

The study showed that 31.5% of smokers intented to quit smoking, 30.8% among Jordanians and 39.8% smong Syrians, which is lower than in a local survey among adults in Amman, Jordan, in 2009-2010 (42%) (4), lower than in India in 2016-2017 (52.2%) (9) and in 2009-2010 (50.9%), and lower than in Kazakhstan (75.9%) (11), and in Malaysia (85.2%) (12). However, the intention to quit prevalence in our study was higher than among older adult smokers in South Korea (26.3%) (13), and among adults in Lebanon (24%) (14). Intensified tobacco control activities are needed in Jordan to increase the intention to quit smoking in the general population.

We found that Syrians were more likely to have intentions to quit smoking than Jordanians, meaning that increased efforts should be made to address Jordanians to promote smoking cessation (18). Some previous research (9, 12, 15) showed an association between other sociodemographic factors, such as age, sex, and education, and intention to quit smoking; however, we did not such associations in this study.

Consistent with previous research (4, 6, 9, 12, 15), we found that history of attempts to quit, exposure to smoking health warnings, and in unadjusted analysis health care advice to quit increased the odds of intention to quit smoking. Health care and anti-tobacco media messaging could be increased, in particular to those with failed quit attempts, so as to increase cessation intentions and eventually successful attempts to quit smoking (10).

Unlike some previous studies (4, 6), we did not find an association between current smokeless tobacco use, heaviness of smoking (daily versus non-daily), life time alcohol use and the intention to quit smoking. An explanation for this finding may be due to the very low prevalence of current smokeless tobacco use (0.2%) and alcohol use (11.6%). Only a few primary health care centres offer free pharmacotherapy and counselling to quit smoking in Jordan, which should be expanded (19).

The study strength is the nationally representative sample of Jordanians and Syrians in Jordan. Study limitations included the cross-sectional design which precludes causative inferences, and some self-reported data, which may have biased responses. Some variables, such as knowledge about the negative health effects of smoking, restrictions of smoking inside the house, and dependence symptoms of smoking, were not assessed in this survey and should be included in further research.

Conclusion

In this national sample of Jordanians and Syrians in Jordan about one in three adults in Jordan intent to quit smoking. Being Syrian, past year smoking quit attempt and having noticed health warnings on cigarette smoking in the newspaper increased the odds of the intention to quit smoking. The anti-tobacco media messages and brief advice to quit should be expanded to increase the quit rate in Jordan.

Acknowledgments

This paper used data from the 2019 Jordan STEPS survey, implemented by the Ministry of Health and Centre for Strategic Studies of the University of Jordan with the support of the World Health Organization.

References

[1] World Health Organization (WHO). Tobacco factsheet, 2019. URL: https://www.who.int/news-room/fact-sheets/detail/tobacco.

[2] Abu-Helalah MA, Alshraideh HA, Al-Serhan AA, Nesheiwat AI, Da'na M, Al-Nawafleh A. Epidemiology, attitudes and perceptions toward cigarettes and hookah smoking amongst adults in Jordan. Environ Health Prev Med 2015;20(6):422-33. doi: 10.1007/s12199-015-0483-1.

[3] Sweis NJ. The economics of tobacco use in Jordan. Chicago, IL: Graduate College, University of Illinois at Chicago, 2013.

[4] Abughosh S, Wu IH, Hawari F, Peters RJ, Yang M, Crutchley R, et al. Predictors of intention to quit cigarette smoking among Jordanian adults. Epidemiology 2011;1:1-7. http://dx.doi.org/10.4172/2161-1165.1000103.

[5] Taylor DH Jr, Hasselblad V, Henley SJ, Thun MJ, Sloan FA. Benefits of smoking cessation for longevity. Am J Public Health 2002;92(6):990-6. doi: 10.2105/ajph.92.6.990. Erratum in: Am J Public Health 2002;92(9):1389.

[6] Karmacharya BM, Fitzpatrick AL, Koju R, Sotodehnia N, Xu DR, Pradhan PMS, et al. Quit intentions and attempts among smokers in sub-urban Nepal: Findings from the Dhulikhel Heart Study. Kathmandu Univ Med J (KUMJ) 2018;16(61): 83-8.

[7] World Bank. Jordan: Overview of tobacco use, tobacco control, legislation and taxation, 2019. URL: https://openknowledge.worldbank.org/handle/10986/31954#:~:text=Jordan%20adopted%20the%20National%20tobacco,by%2030%20percent%20by%202025.

[8] World Health Organization (WHO). WHO report on the global tobacco epidemic, 2021 Country profile Jordan. URL: https://cdn.who.int/media/docs/default-source/country-profiles/tobacco/who_rgte_2021_jordan.pdf?sfvrsn=d182273e_5&download=true.

[9] Kar SS, Sivanantham P, Rehman T, Chinnakali P, Thiagarajan S. Willingness to quit tobacco and its correlates among Indian tobacco users. Findings from the Global Adult Tobacco Survey India, 2016-17. J Postgrad Med 2020;66(3):141-8. doi: 10.4103/jpgm.JPGM_408_19.

[10] Reddy MM, Kanungo S, Naik BN, Kar SS. Willingness to quit tobacco smoking and its correlates among Indian smokers: Findings from Global Adult Tobacco Survey India, 2009-2010. J Fam Med Prim Care 2018;7(6):1353-60. doi: 10.4103/jfmpc.jfmpc_169_18.

[11] Wang Q, Mati K. Intention to quit among smokers in Kazakhstan: Data from 2014 Global Adult Tobacco Survey. J Epidemiol Glob Health 2019;9(1):23-8. doi: 10.2991/jegh.k.190212.002.

[12] Hasan SI, Kaai SC, Amer Nordin AS, Mohd Hairi F, Danaee M, Yee A, et al. Who are more likely to have quit intentions among Malaysian adult smokers? Findings from the 2020 ITC Malaysia Survey. Int J Environ Res Public Health 2022;19(5):3035. doi: 10.3390/ijerph19053035.

[13] Lee I, Park YS, Kim JH, Han SH. Factors associated with the intention to quit smoking in elderly Korean men: The Korea National Health and Nutrition Examination Survey 2010-2015. Korean J Fam Med 2020;41(4):237-42. doi: 10.4082/kjfm.18.0124.

[14] Chaaya M, Nakkash R, Saab D, Kadi L, Afifi R. Effect of tobacco control policies on intention to quit smoking cigarettes: A study from Beirut, Lebanon. Tob Induc Dis 2019;17:63. doi: 10.18332/tid/111128.

[15] Iken O, Cadmus E, Ahmed B. Correlates of quit intentions among current Nigerian smokers: Evidence from the 2012 Global Adult Tobacco Surveys (GATS). Tob Prev Cessat 2020;6:13. doi: 10.18332/tpc/115168.

[16] World Health Organization (WHO). STEPwise approach to surveillance (STEPS), 2018. URL: https://www.who.int/ncds/surveillance/steps/en/.

[17] Ministry of Health, Jordan National Stepwise Survey (STEPs) for Noncommunicable Diseases Risk Factors 2019. URL: https://extranet.who.int/ncdsmicrodata/index.php/catalog/853/download/6010.

[18] Phiri MM, Summers AD, Kress AC, de Quevedo IG, Caraballo R, Twentyman E. Demographic characteristics associated with awareness of cigarette health warnings and thinking about quitting among current adult cigarette smokers in Zambia, 2017. Tob Prev Cessat 2022;8:05. doi: 10.18332/tpc/144772.

[19] Saqf el Hait S, Basheti I. Narrative review of smoking cessation practices in Jordan. J Pharm Clin Res 2017;2(4):555591. doi: 10.19080/JPCR.2017.02.555591.

Chapter 5

Prevalence and correlates of non-communicable disease risk factors among Jordanian and Syrian adults in Jordan

Karl Peltzer[*]**, PhD**

Department of Psychology, University of the Free State, Bloemfontein, South Africa
Department of Psychology, College of Medical and Health Science, Asia University, Taichung, Taiwan

Abstract

In this chapter we aimed to estimate the prevalence and associated factors of behavioural and biological non-communicable disease (NCD) risk factors among adults in Jordan in 2019. National data were analysed from 5,713 adults (50.9% Jordanians and 49.1% Syrian) aged 18 to 69 years (mean 36.7) who participated in the cross-sectional "2019 Jordan STEPS survey." The prevalence of inadequate fruit and vegetable intake was 86.4%, followed by dyslipidaemia (81.6%), central obesity (56.5%), current smoking (40.3%), low physical activity (30.4%), hypertension (25.5%), sedentary behaviour (23.5%) and diabetes (7.5%). In adjusted logistic regression analysis, male sex (AOR: 8.31, 95% CI: 6.20-11.15), and Jordanian (AOR: 2.15, 95% CI: 1.61-2.89) were positively associated and older age (60-69 years) (AOR: 0.38, 95% CI: 0.22-0.67), higher education (≥12 years) (AOR: 0.63, 95% CI: 0.43-0.93) and higher monthly household income (AOR: 0.69, 95% CI: 0.48-1.00) were negatively associated with current smoking. Older age (60-69 years) (AOR: 0.50, 95% CI: 0.30-0.88), higher household income (AOR: 0.27, 95% CI: 0.17-0.45), and Jordanian (AOR: 0.61, 95% CI: 0.42-0.89) were

[*] ***Correspondence:*** Professor Karl Peltzer, Department of Psychology, University of the Free State, PO Box 339 (40), Bloemfontein 9300, South Africa. Email: kfpeltzer@gmail.com.

In: Non-Communicable Diseases
Editor: Joav Merrick
ISBN: 979-8-89113-514-7

inversely associated with insufficient fruit and vegetable intake. Older age (60-69 years) was positively associated with central obesity, hypertension, diabetes, and dyslipidaemia. Male sex (AOR: 0.26, 95% CI: 0.19-0.36) was negatively associated with central obesity, and having three or four health risk behaviours (AOR: 2.07, 95% CI: 1.17-3.65) was positively associated with dyslipidaemia. A high prevalence and associated factors of behavioural and biological risk factors of NCD were identified that can assist in planning interventions.

Introduction

More than 85% of premature deaths from noncommunicable diseases (NCDs) occur in lower resourced countries (1). In Jordan, an upper middle-income country in the eastern Mediterranean, NCDs contribute to 78% mortality in 2018 (2). NCD death is mainly caused by "cardiovascular diseases, cancers, respiratory diseases, and diabetes" (1). Behavioural risk behaviours, such as smoking, hazardous alcohol use, sedentary behaviour and unhealthy diets, significantly increase the risk of NCD mortality (1). The Eastern Mediterranean region is experiencing a rapid increase in NCDs, and it is "crucial to have a careful understanding of the local drivers of NCDs" (3). Against this backdrop, recent national community-based information on behavioural and biological NCD risk factors in Jordan is needed.

Among community-dwelling Syrians in northern Jordan in 2016, the self-reported prevalence of hypertension was 14.0%, diabetes 9.2% and cardiovascular conditions 5.7% (4). In a medical examination sub-sample of the 2007 "Jordan Behavioral Risk Factor Surveillance Survey", 36.0% had obesity, 29.8% hypertension, 19.5% diabetes, and 13.9% high cholesterol (5). In a cross-sectional in five regional governorates of Jordan (18–79 years), current smoking was among men 59.1% and among women 23.3% (6). In a population ($\geq$25 years) in northern Jordan in 2002, the prevalence of obesity was 53.1% among women and 28.1% among men 7), and in northern Jordan, 75.7% had dyslipidaemia ($\geq$1 abnormal lipid level) (8). The prevalence of population diabetes ($\geq$25 years) in Jordan increased from 13.0% in 1994 to 23.7% in 2017 (9). In outpatient relatives (N=340) in Jordan, the prevalence of low physical activity was 50.3% (10).

In a national STEPS survey in Lebanon, the prevalence of current smoking was 38.0% (among Lebanese)/31.1% (among Syrian refugees), inadequate fruit and vegetable intake 73.4%/93.2% and low physical activity 61.0% (among Lebanese)/61.7% (among Syrian refugees) (11). The prevalence of hypertension in this survey in Lebanon was 35.3% (among Lebanese)/32.8% (among Syrian refugees), obesity 27.0%/28.6%, diabetes 10.5%/9.4%, and raised total cholesterol 65.4%/48.8% (11). In the Kenya STEPS survey in 2015, 10.1% had high blood total cholesterol, 80.3% low physical activity, 99.8% had inadequate fruit and vegetable intake, 22.4% obesity, 24.8% hypertension, 2.6% diabetes, 10.2% smoking, and 13.8% harmful alcohol use (12). In the Nepal STEPS survey in 2013, the prevalence of current smoking was 18.5%, overweight/obesity 21.4%, hypertension 25.7%, insufficient fruit/vegetable consumption 98.9%, low physical activity 3.4%, raised total cholesterol 22.6%, and diabetes 3.6% (13). In Bolivia, the prevalence of current smoking was 11.6%, low physical activity 64.8%, central obesity 54.1%, elevated blood pressure 17.5% and inadequate fruit and vegetable intake 76.7% (14).

As previously reviewed (15), factors associated with NCD risk factors include currently married, sex, older age, geographic region, urban residence, educational status, and higher economic level. The study aimed to estimate the prevalence and associated factors of behavioural and biological NCD among adults in Jordan in 2019.

Our study

National cross-sectional data from the 2019 Jordan STEPS survey (response rate 63-95%) (16, 17) were analysed. Following STEPS methodology:

> "Socio-demographic and behavioural information was collected in Step 1. Physical measurements such as height, weight, and blood pressure were collected in Step 2. Biochemical measurements were collected to assess blood glucose and cholesterol levels in Step 3. A multi-stage stratified sampling process was carried out to randomly select participants from the target population of adult Jordanians and Syrians. One individual within the age range of the survey (18-69 years) was selected per household. Ethics approval was provided by the Ethics Committee of the Jordan Ministry of Health for Scientific Research, and written informed consent was obtained from all participants." (16, 17)

Our measures

Outcome variables: NCD risk factors

Behavioural NCD risk factors included current smoking, low physical activity and sedentary behaviour (≥8 hrs/day) based on the "Global Physical Activity Questionnaire" (19) and fruit/vegetable intake (<5 servings/day) (17).

Biological NCD risk factors. Central obesity ("waist circumference ≥94 cm in men, ≥80 cm in women") (20); *Diabetes*: "fasting plasma glucose levels >=7.0 mmol/L (≥126 mg/dl); or using insulin or oral hypoglycaemic drugs." (18); *Hypertension/raised blood pressure* (BP): "systolic BP ≥140 mm Hg and/or diastolic BP ≥90 mm Hg or where the participant is currently on antihypertensive medication." (21) *Dyslipidaemia* was classified (22) as:

> "being on antilipidemic medication or having one or more of the following: elevated total cholesterol (TC): ≥5.17 mmol/l (200 mg/dl), high triglycerides (TG): ≥1.70 mmol/l (150 mg/dl), low high-density lipoprotein cholesterol (HDL-C): female ≤1.29 mmol/l; ≤male 1.03 (<50 mg/dl in women, <40 mg/dl in men) and high low-density lipoprotein cholesterol (LDL-C): ≥3.36 mmol/l (130 mg/dl)"

The exposure variables consisted of education, sex, age, region, nationality, residence, and monthly household income (in Jordanian Dinar (JD) ("1st June 2019: $1 *USD* = JD 0.709") (17). In addition, an index of health risk behaviour (summed sedentary behaviour, low physical activity, inadequate fruit and vegetable intake, and current smoking) was formed and grouped into 0-1, 2, and 3 or for health risk behaviours.

All statistical analyses were conducted with "STATA software version 14.0 (Stata Corporation, College Station, TX, USA)," considering sampling weights. Descriptive statistics are used to describe NCD risk factors. Logistic regressions were used to assess the associations between sociodemographic and health factors and specific NCD risk factors. Linear regressions were used to assess the predictors of multiple NCD risk factors. P-values <0.05 were considered significant.

Our findings

The sample included 5,713 adults (50.9% Jordanians and 49.1% Syrians) aged 18 to 69 years (mean 36.7, SD=14.0). Majority were females (61.4%), living in the central region (56.5%) and resided in urban areas (81.3%). Further details are provided in Table 1.

Table 1. Sample characteristics, Jordan, 2019

Variable	Subcategory	Jordanian N (%[a])	Syrian N (%[a])	All N (%[a])
Total		2910 (50.9)	2803 (49.1)	5713
Age (years)	18-29	724 (24.9)	878 (31.3)	1602 (28.0)
	30-44	939 (32.3)	1207 (43.1)	2146 (37.6)
	45-59	819 (28.1)	520 (18.6)	1339 (23.4)
	60-69	428 (14.7)	198 (7.1)	626 (11.0)
Gender	Female	1712 (58.8)	1798 (64.1)	3510 (61.4)
	Male	1198 (41.2)	1005 (35.9_	2203 (38.6)
Education (in years)	0-6	453 (15.6)	1122 (40.0)	1575 (27.6)
	7-11	863 (29.7)	1091 (38.9)	1954 (34.2)
	≥12	1594 (54.8)	590 (21.0)	2184 (38.2)
Monthly household income (in Jordanian Dinar)	<200	346 (12.8)	928 (36.6)	1274 (24.3)
	200-349	931 (34.4)	1199 (47.2)	2130 (40.6)
	≥350	1428 (52.8)	411 (16.2)	1839 (35.1)
Marital status	Not married	949 (32.7)	633 (22.6)	1582 (27.7)
	Married	1956 (67.3)	2169 (77.4)	4125 (72.3)
Residence	Rural	567 (19.5)	501 (17.9)	2068 (18.7)
	Urban	2343 (80.5)	2302 (82.1)	4645 (81.3)
Region	Center	1708 (58.7)	1521 (54.3)	3229 (56.5)
	North	904 (31.1)	1282 (45.7)	2186 (38.3)
	South	298 (10.2)	---	298 (5.2)

[a]Unweighted.

NCD risk factors

The prevalence of inadequate fruit/vegetable intake was 86.4%, followed by dyslipidaemia (81.6%), central obesity (56.5%), current smoking (40.3%), low physical activity (30.4%), hypertension (25.5%), sedentary behaviour (23.5%), and diabetes (7.5%). In total 80.6% of participants had three or more of the eight assessed NCD risk factors (see Table 2).

Associations with behavioural NCD risk factors
In multivariable regression model, male sex (AOR: 8.31, 95% CI: 6.20-11.15), and being Jordanian (AOR: 2.15, 95% CI: 1.61-2.89) were positively, and older age (60-69 years) (AOR: 0.38, 95% CI: 0.22-0.67), higher education (≥12 years) (AOR: 0.63, 95% CI: 0.43-0.93) and having a monthly household income of 200-349 Jordanian Dinars (JD) (AOR: 0.69, 95% CI: 0.48-1.00) were negatively associated with current smoking. Older age (60-69 years) (AOR: 0.50, 95% CI: 0.30-0.88), higher household income (≥350 JD) (AOR: 0.27, 95% CI: 0.17-0.45), and being Jordanian (AOR: 0.61, 95% CI: 0.42-0.89) were inversely associated with insufficient fruit and vegetable intake. Compared to adults 18-29 years of age, older adults (60-69 years) (AOR: 3.08, 95% CI: 1.99-4.75) had three times higher odds of low physical activity. Older age (60-69 years) (AOR: 2.65, 95% CI: 1.59-3.81), male sex (AOR: 1.71, 95% CI: 1.30-2.14), living in the Northern region of the country (AOR: 1.52, 95% CI: 1.10-2.11) were positively and higher education (≥12 years) (AOR: 0.69, 95% CI: 0.49-0.97) was negatively associated with sedentary behaviour (see Table 3).

Associations with biological NCD risk factors
In adjusted logistic regression analysis, older age (60-69 years) was positively associated with central obesity (AOR: 15.12, 95% CI: 8.75-26.11), hypertension (AOR: 11.06, 95% CI: 6.50-18.84), diabetes (AOR: 15.19, 95% CI: 5.14-44.92) and dyslipidaemia (AOR: 2.08, 95% CI: 1.15-3.76). Male sex (AOR: 0.26, 95% CI: 0.19-0.36) was negatively and married (AOR: 1.44, 95% CI: 1.01-2.05) was positively associated with central obesity. Having three or four health risk behaviours (AOR: 2.07, 95% CI: 1.17-3.65) was positively associated with dyslipidaemia (see Table 4).

Linear regression with eight NCD risk factors
In adjusted linear regression analysis, in both sexes, older age (60-69 years) (Adjusted Exp Coef.: 3.78, 95% CI: 2.71-5.28), male sex (A Exp Coef.: 1.40, 95% CI: 1.20-1.63), being Jordanian (A Exp Coef.: 1.35, 95% CI: 1.15-1.57) were positively and higher education (A Exp Coef.: 0.65, 95% CI: 0.51-0.81) was negatively associated with a higher degree of NCD risk factors. Additionally, in gender stratified analysis, among men urban residence (A Exp Coef.: 1.46, 95% CI: 1.05-2.02) was postiviely and among women married (A Exp Coef.: 0.75, 95% CI: 0.62-0.91) was negatively associated with a higher degree of risk factors for NCD (see Table 5).

Table 2. Distribution of behavioural and biological non-communicable risk factors in weighted percent

Variable	Subcategory	Current smoking	Inadequate fruit and vegetable intake	Low physical activity	Sedentary behaviour	Central obesity	Hypertension	Diabetes	Dyslipidaemia
Total		40.3	86.4	30.4	23.5	56.5	25.5	7.5	81.6
Age (years)	18-29	42.4	89.5	24.3	23.0	29.7	9.7	2.4	75.4
	30-44	44.0	86.6	27.2	18.1	64.1	22.6	4.1	82.4
	45-59	35.0	83.3	39.5	26.9	81.0	46.9	18.0	86.8
	60-69	25.9	78.7	50.9	42.1	87.0	60.8	23.6	88.5
Gender	Female	18.2	86.7	30.4	18.6	71.3	26.6	6.7	82.3
	Male	62.1	86.1	30.3	28.4	42.5	24.4	8.3	80.8
Education (in years)	0-6	35.4	88.0	34.6	31.6	73.0	42.0	14.5	83.8
	7-11	48.8	89.7	29.3	22.3	54.5	23.7	8.1	84.4
	≥12	35.7	83.6	29.9	22.0	53.4	21.9	5.1	78.9
Monthly household income (in Jordanian Dinar)	<200	40.4	95.2	29.2	22.8	60.3	30.0	8.8	85.2
	200-349	38.4	88.2	30.7	25.2	55.5	25.5	7.7	81.9
	≥350	42.7	82.6	29.6	22.6	55.6	23.9	6.6	80.5
Marital status	Not married	44.3	89.3	25.6	24.1	38.3	15.7	5.2	78.7
	Married	37.5	84.4	33.5	23.1	69.1	31.9	9.1	83.2
Nationality	Syrian	31.3	93.6	27.8	22.0	54.0	20.7	4.7	77.8
	Jordanian	41.3	85.5	30.7	23.7	56.8	26.0	7.9	82.0
Residence	Rural	36.9	85.1	29.1	26.6	53.9	26.2	6.5	82.0
	Urban	40.9	86.6	30.6	22.9	57.0	25.3	7.7	81.5
Region	Center	41.4	87.1	30.8	19.5	57.0	26.0	8.2	80.8
	North	36.6	86.0	29.4	27.0	56.8	24.8	6.1	82.8
	South	47.8	83.4	31.6	35.3	51.9	24.9	9.0	82.0

Table 3. Associations with behavioural non-communicable disease risk factors

Variable	Subcategory	Current smoking	Insufficient fruit/ vegetable intake	Low physical activity	Sedentary behaviour
		AOR (95% CI)	AOR (95% CI)	AOR (95% CI)	AOR (95% CI)
Age (years)	18-29	1 (Reference)	1 (Reference)	1 (Reference)	1 (Reference)
	30-44	1.50 (1.00, 2.25)*	0.91 (0.54, 1.55)	1.06 (0.72, 1.55)	0.84 (0.58, 1.22)
	45-59	0.90 (0.59, 1.36)	0.73 (0,42, 1.27)	1.79 (1.25, 2.56)***	1.42 (0.98, 2.07)
	60-69	0.38 (0.22, 0.67)***	0.50 (0.30, 0.88)*	3.08 (1.99, 4.75)***	2.65 (1.59, 3.81)***
Gender	Female	1 (Reference)	1 (Reference)	1 (Reference)	1 (Reference)
	Male	8.31 (6.20, 11.15)***	0.98 (0.69, 1.31)	0.93 (0.72, 1.20)	1.71 (1.30, 2.24)**
Education (in years)	0-6	1 (Reference)	1 (Reference)	1 (Reference)	1 (Reference)
	7-11	1.15 (0.80, 1.67)	1.25 (0.79, 1.99)	0.94 (0.68, 1.31)	0.73 (0.52, 1.04)
	≥12	0.63 (0.43, 0.93)*	0.78 (0.51, 1.19)	0.97 (0.71, 1.32)	0.69 (0.49, 0.97)*
Monthly household income (in Jordanian Dinar)	<200	1 (Reference)	1 (Reference)	1 (Reference)	1 (Reference)
	200-349	0.69 (0.48, 1.00)*	0.40 (0.24, 0.67)***	1.09 (0.76, 1.58)	1.19 (0.85, 1.68)
	≥350	0.82 (0.58, 1.17)	0.27 (0.17, 0.45)***	1.06 (0.74, 1.53)	1.07 (0.74, 1.55)
Marital status	Not married	1 (Reference)	1 (Reference)	1 (Reference)	1 (Reference)
	Married	0.84 (0.60, 1.17)	0.70 (0.45, 1.07)	1.19 (0.86, 1.65)	0.87 (0.62, 1.23)
Nationality	Syrian	1 (Reference)	1 (Reference)	1 (Reference)	1 (Reference)
	Jordanian	2.15 (1.61, 2.89)***	0.61 (0.42, 0.89)*	1.09 (0.83, 1.41)	1.02 (0.76, 1.36)
Residence	Rural	1 (Reference)	1 (Reference)	1 (Reference)	1 (Reference)
	Urban	1.38 (0.96, 2.00)	1.11 (0.76, 1.62)	1.10 (0.75, 1.60)	0.87 (0.60, 1.27)
Region	Center	1 (Reference)	1 (Reference)	1 (Reference)	1 (Reference)
	North	0.77 (0.57, 1.04)	0.83 (0.56, 1.21)	1.04 (0.79, 1.37)	1.52 (1.10, 2.11)*
	South	0.78 (0.51, 1.20)	0.88 (0.53, 1.43)	1.05 (0.68, 1.64)	1.83 (1.14, 2.94)

***$p < 0.001$; **$p < 0.01$; *$p < 0.05$; AOR = Adjusted Odds Ratio; CI = Confidence Interval.

Table 4. Associations with biological non-communicable disease risk factors

Variable	Subcategory	Central obesity	Hypertension	Diabetes	Dyslipidaemia
		AOR (95% CI)	AOR (95% CI)	AOR (95% CI)	AOR (95% CI)
Age (years)	18-29	1 (Reference)	1 (Reference)	1 (Reference)	1 (Reference)
	30-44	3.45 (2.30, 5.19)***	2.44 (1.48, 4.02)***	2.71 (0.90, 8.09)	1.39 (0.89, 2.17)
	45-59	9.04 (5.80, 14.10)***	7.02 (4.23, 11.65)***	13.65 (5.02, 37.11)***	2.09 (1.27, 3.45)**
	60-69	15.12 (8.75, 26.11)***	11.06 (6.50, 18.84)***	15.19 (5.14, 44.92)***	2.08 (1.15, 3.76)*
Gender	Female	1 (Reference)	1 (Reference)	1 (Reference)	1 (Reference)
	Male	0.26 (0.19, 0.36)***	0.89 (0.65, 1.21)	1.09 (0.70, 1.69)	0.80 (0.55, 1.17)
Education (in years)	0-6	1 (Reference)	1 (Reference)	1 (Reference)	1 (Reference)
	7-11	0.90 (0.58, 1.39)	0.82 (0.56, 1.20)	1.05 (0.64, 1.72)	1.49 (0.86, 2.57)
	≥12	0.75 (0.48, 1.16)	0.70 (0.47, 1.05)	0.52 (0.30, 0.88)	0.91 (0.55, 1.52)
Monthly household income (in Jordanian Dinar)	<200	1 (Reference)	1 (Reference)	1 (Reference)	1 (Reference)
	200-349	0.88 (0.58, 1.32)	0.85 (0.57, 1.27)	1.10 (0.60, 1.71)	0.78 (0.49, 1.24)
	≥350	1.08 (0.70, 1.67)	0.82 (0.54, 1.26)	0.97 (0.57, 1.66)	0.79 (0.50, 1.25)
Marital status	Not married	1 (Reference)	1 (Reference)	1 (Reference)	1 (Reference)
	Married	1.44 (1.01, 2.05)*	1.20 (0.83, 1.74)	0.77 (0.47, 1.26)	0.93 (0.61, 1.41)
Nationality	Syrian	1 (Reference)	1 (Reference)	1 (Reference)	1 (Reference)
	Jordanian	1.17 (0.87, 1.56)	1.32 (0.96, 1.80)	1.37 (0.90, 2.07)	1.33 (0.93, 1.91)
Residence	Rural	1 (Reference)	1 (Reference)	1 (Reference)	1 (Reference)
	Urban	1.08 (0.72, 1.64)	0.91 (0.66, 1.26)	1.20 (0.67, 2.16)	1.01 (0.63, 1.63)
Region	Center	1 (Reference)	1 (Reference)	1 (Reference)	1 (Reference)
	North	1.15 (0.83, 1.58)	0.99 (0.75, 1.32)	0.82 (0.52, 1.31)	1.16 (0.76, 1.75)
	South	1.10 (0.62, 1.95)	0.96 (0.53, 1.73)	1.22 (0.61, 2.45)	1.45 (0.53, 3.95)
Health risk behaviour	0-1	1 (Reference)	1 (Reference)	1 (Reference)	1 (Reference)
	2	0.93 (0.67, 1.29)	1.09 (0.80, 1.48)	1.01 (0.61, 1.66)	1.22 (0.81, 1.83)
	3-4	0.91 (0.60, 1.38)	1.33 (0.90, 1.96)	1.67 (0.93, 3.02)	2.07 (1.17, 3.65)*

***$p < 0.001$; **$p < 0.01$; *$p < 0.05$; AOR = Adjusted Odds Ratio; CI = Confidence Interval.

Table 5. Linear regression with eight NCD risk factors

Variable	Subcategory	Both sexes	Men	Women
		Adjusted Exp (Coef.) (95% CI)	Adjusted Exp (Coef.) (95% CI)	Adjusted Exp (Coef.) (95% CI)
Age (years)	18-29	Reference	Reference	Reference
	30-44	1.45 (1.16, 1.81)***	1.58 (1.02, 2.44)*	1.21 (0.97, 1.52)
	45-59	2.95 (2.32, 3.75)***	2.79 (1.71, 4.56)***	2.61 (2.03, 3.36)***
	60-69	3.78 (2.71, 5.28)***	3.22 (1.73, 5.98)***	3.47 (2.51, 4.79)***
Gender	Female	Reference	---	---
	Male	1.40 (1.20, 1.63)***		
Education (in years)	0-6	Reference	Reference	Reference
	7-11	0.98 (0.77, 1.25)	1.17 (0.79, 1.75)	0.84 (0.66, 1.08)
	≥12	0.65 (0.51, 0.81)***	0.66 (0.45, 0.98)*	0.61 (0.47, 0.79)***
Monthly household income (in Jordanian Dinar)	<200	Reference	Reference	Reference
	200-349	0.91 (0.74, 1.12)	0.79 (0.56, 1.11)	1.02 (0.81, 1.29)
	≥350	0.85 (0.69, 1.05)	0.89 (0.63, 1.24)	0.89 (0.69, 1.14)
Marital status	Not married	Reference	Reference	Reference
	Married	0.96 (0.79, 1.16)	1.42 (0.95, 2.13)	0.75 (0.62, 0.91)**
Nationality	Syrian	Reference	Reference	Reference
	Jordanian	1.35 (1.15, 1.57)***	1.60 (1.24, 2.07)***	1.20 (1.00, 1.43)*
Residence	Rural	Reference	Reference	Reference
	Urban	1.18 (0.97, 1.43)	1.46 (1.05, 2.02)*	0.98 (0.77, 1.25)
Region	Center	Reference	Reference	Reference
	North	1.00 (0.85, 1.19)	1.01 (0.76, 1.35)	0.91 (0.77, 1.08)
	South	1.04 (0.73, 1.47)	1.07 (0.62, 1.86)	0.93 (0.71, 1.22)

Exp (Coef.) = Exponentiated Coefficients, CI = Confidence Interval; ***$p < 0.001$; **$p < 0.01$; *$p < 0.05$.

Discussion

The study found in a national sample of Jordanians and Syrians (18-69 years) in Jordan that the four most prevalent NCD risk factors were insufficient fruit/vegetable intake (86.4%), dyslipidaemia (81.6%), central obesity (56.5%) and current smoking (40.3%). Similar results were found in the Lebanese survey, with inadequate fruit and vegetable intake (73.4%/93.2%), followed by raised total cholesterol (65.4%/48.8%), overweight/obesity (73.4%/73.4%), and current smoking (38.0% among Lebanese/31.1% among Syrian refugees) (11). The high prevalence of insufficient fruit/vegetable consumption (86.4%) was similar to the Jordan STEPS 2007 survey (85.8%) (23), lower than in Kenya (99.8%) (12), Nepal (98.9%] (13), and higher than in Bolivia (76.7%) (14). The prevalence of current smoking (40.3%) was similar to a study in five regional governorates of Jordan (59.1% among men and 23.3% among women) (6), and the Jordan Global Adult Tobacco Survey (GATS) in 2011 (42.2%) (24) but was much higher than in Kenya (10.2%) (12), in Nepal (18.5%) (13) and in Bolivia (11.6%) (14). Implementing and strengthening tobacco control policies are urgently needed in Jordan (17), including increases in exercise tax and the price of tobacco products (24). The high prevalence of dyslipidaemia (81.6%) was similar to a study in northern Jordan (75.7%) (8).

The prevalence of low physical activity (30.4%) was lower than in relatives of outpatients in Jordan (50.3%) (10), lower than in Kenya (80.3%) and Bolivia (64.8%) (14), but higher than in Nepal (3.4%) (13). The prevalence of hypertension (25.5%) was the same as in the Jordan STEPS survey in 2007 (25.5%) (23), a little lower than in a medical examination subsample of the 2007 "Jordan Behavioral Risk Factor Surveillance Survey" (29.8%) (5), similar to Kenya (24.8%) (12), Nepal (25.7%) (13) and higher than in Bolivia (17.5%) (14). The prevalence of diabetes (7.5%) was lower than previous estimates in Jordan, 19.5% in the 2007 "Jordan Behavioral Risk Factor Surveillance Survey" (5), and 23.7% in population estimates in 2017 (9), but higher than in Kenya (2.6%) (12), and in Nepal (3.6%) (13).

The study found that sociodemographic factors (male sex, Jordanian, younger age, and lower education) increased the chances of current smoking. Older age, higher household income, and being Jordanian were protective against insufficient fruit and vegetable intake. Older age increased the odds of low physical activity and sedentary behaviour. Syrians had a higher prevalence of inadequate fruit and vegetable intake than Jordanians. It is possible that Syrians, as being refugees, have less access to fruits and vegetables. Interventions should be geared towards increasing fruit and vegetable intake, in particular with Syrians. The Jordan STEPS survey team (17) recommends to:

> "Reduce physical inactivity through the implementation of the WHO Global Strategy on Diet, Physical Activity and Health. Increase public awareness of the importance and impact of physical activity on health by implementing community-wide public awareness campaigns through mass media and community-based education to support behavioural change."

In terms of biological NCD risk factors older age was positively associated with central obesity, hypertension, diabetes, and dyslipidaemia. Male sex was negatively and married was positively associated with central obesity. Having three or four health risk behaviours was positively associated with dyslipidaemia. Similarly, health risk behaviours increased the risk of cardiovascular risk factors in Chile (25). Central obesity was higher in women than in men, while current smoking and sedentary behaviour were higher in men than in women. Similar results were found in the Kenya STEPS survey (12). The higher prevalence of obesity in women may be attributed to biological, comorbidity and lifestyle factors (7,26). In targeting interventions these sex differences should be taken into consideration (17). The Jordan STEPS survey team (17) recommends:

> "Increasing awareness of the community on the importance of early detection for raised blood pressure, diabetes and hyperlipidemia through ensuring regular and annual mass screening under the supervision of the MOH. Moreover, have proper control of those diagnosed by ensuring the provision of essential medications and treatment."

Regarding the eight NCD risk factors evaluated, male sex, older age, Jordanian, lower education, and among men urban residence were associated with a higher number of NCD risk factors. Regarding increasing age, early detection, especially among males, those with lower education, Jordanians, and men in urban areas, should be targeted to prevent a buildup of NCD risk factors in Jordan.

The study strength is the nationally representative sample of Jordanians and Syrians in Jordan. Study limitations included the cross-sectional design which precludes causative inferences, and some self-reported data, which may been been biased. Furthermore, there was a low study response rate for the biochemical measures (63%).

Conclusion

In this national sample of Jordanians and Syrians in Syria four in five participants had three or more risk factors for NCD. Older age, male sex, being Jordanian and urban residence increased the risk for a higher degree of NCD risk factors. Increased multisectoral NCD risk reduction strategies are needed in Jordan.

Acknowledgments

This paper uses data from the 2019 Jordan STEPS survey, implemented by the Ministry of Health and Centre for Strategic Studies of the University of Jordan with the support of the World Health Organization.

References

[1] World Health Organization (WHO). Noncommunicable diseases, 2018. URL: https://www.who.int/news-room/fact-sheets/detail/noncommunicable-diseases.

[2] World Health Organization (WHO). Jordan: Noncommunicable Diseases (NCD) Country Profiles, 2018. URL: https://www.who.int/nmh/countries/jor_en.pdf.

[3] World Health Organization (WHO). Non-communicable diseases. URL: http://www.emro.who.int/noncommunicable-diseases/publications/burden-of-noncommunicable-diseases-in-the-eastern-mediterranean-region.html.

[4] Rehr M, Shoaib M, Ellithy S, Okour S, Ariti C, Ait-Bouziad I, et al. Prevalence of non-communicable diseases and access to care among non-camp Syrian refugees in northern Jordan. Confl Health 2018;12:33. doi: 10.1186/s13031-018-0168-7.

[5] Al-Nsour M, Zindah M, Belbeisi A, Hadaddin R, Brown DW, Walke H. Prevalence of selected chronic, noncommunicable disease risk factors in Jordan: results of the 2007 Jordan Behavioral Risk Factor Surveillance Survey. Prev Chronic Dis 2012;9:E25.

[6] Abu-Helalah MA, Alshraideh HA, Al-Serhan AA, Nesheiwat AI, Da'na M, Al-Nawafleh A. Epidemiology, attitudes and perceptions toward cigarettes and hookah smoking amongst adults in Jordan. Environ Health Prev Med 2015;20(6):422-33. doi: 10.1007/s12199-015-0483-1.

[7] Khader Y, Batieha A, Ajlouni H, El-Khateeb M, Ajlouni K. Obesity in Jordan: Prevalence, associated factors, comorbidities, and change in prevalence over ten years. Metab Syndr Relat Disord 2008;6(2):113-20. doi: 10.1089/met.2007.0030.

[8] Khader YS, Batieha A, El-Khateeb M, Al Omari M, Ajlouni K. Prevalence of dyslipidemia and its associated factors among Jordanian adults. J Clin Lipidol 2010;4(1):53-8. doi: 10.1016/j.jacl.2009.12.004.

[9] Ajlouni K, Batieha A, Jaddou H, Khader Y, Abdo N, El-Khateeb M, et al. Time trends in diabetes mellitus in Jordan between 1994 and 2017. Diabet Med 2019;36(9):1176-1182. doi: 10.1111/dme.13894.

[10] Bawadi HA, Khader YS, Haroun TF, Al-Omari M, Tayyem RF. The association between periodontal disease, physical activity and healthy diet among adults in Jordan. J Periodontal Res 2011;46(1):74-81. doi: 10.1111/j.1600-0765.2010.01314.x.

[11] Mansour Z, Said R, Dbaibo H, Mrad P, Torossian L, Rady A, et al. Non-communicable diseases in Lebanon: results from World Health Organization STEPS survey 2017. Public Health 2020;187:120-6. doi: 10.1016/j.puhe.2020.08.014.

[12] Wekesah FM, Nyanjau L, Kibachio J, Mutua MK, Mohamed SF, Grobbee DE, et al. Individual and household level factors associated with presence of multiple non-communicable disease risk factors in Kenyan adults. BMC Public Health 2018;18(Suppl 3):1220. doi:10.1186/s12889-018-6055-8

[13] Aryal KK, Mehata S, Neupane S, Vaidya A, Dhimal M, Dhakal P, et al. The burden and determinants of non communicable diseases risk factors in Nepal: Findings from a Nationwide STEPS Survey. PLoS One 2015;10(8):e0134834. doi:10.1371/journal.pone.0134834.

[14] Mamani-Ortiz Y, San Sebastián M, Armaza AX, Luizaga JM, Illanes DE, Ferrel M, Mosquera PA. Prevalence and determinants of cardiovascular disease risk factors using the WHO STEPS approach in Cochabamba, Bolivia. BMC Public Health 2019;19(1):786. doi: 10.1186/s12889-019-7064-y.

[15] Pengpid S, Peltzer K. Prevalence and correlates of multiple non-communicable disease risk factors among adults in Zambia: results of the first national STEPS survey in 2017. Pan Afr Med J 2020;37:265. doi: 10.11604/pamj.2020.37.265.25038.

[16] World Health Organization (WHO). STEPwise approach to surveillance (STEPS), 2018. URL: https://www.who.int/ncds/surveillance/steps/en/.

[17] Ministry of Health, Jordan National Stepwise Survey (STEPs) for Noncommunicable Diseases risk factors 2019. URL: https://extranet.who.int/ncdsmicrodata/index.php/catalog/853/download/6010.

[18] World Health Organization (WHO). WHO STEPS surveillance manual. URL: https://www.who.int/ncds/surveillance/steps/STEPS_Manual.pdf.

[19] Armstrong T, Bull F. Development of the World Health Organization Global Physical Activity Questionnaire (GPAQ). J Public Health 2006;14:66–70.

[20] Harvard School of Public Health. Abdominal obesity measurement guidelines for different ethnic groups, 2020. URL: https://www.hsph.harvard.edu/obesity-prevention-source/waist-circumference-guidelines-for-different-ethnic-groups/ .

[21] Chobanian AV, Bakris GL, Black HR, Cushman WC, Green LA, Izzo JL et al. Seventh report of the Joint National Committee of Prevention, Detection, Evaluation, and Treatment of High Blood Pressure. Hypertension 2003;42(6):1206–52. http://dx.doi.org/10.1161/01.HYP.0000107251.49515.c2

[22] Expert Panel on Detection, Evaluation, and Treatment of High Blood Cholesterol in Adults. Executive Summary of The Third Report of The National Cholesterol

Education Program (NCEP) Expert Panel on Detection, Evaluation, and Treatment of High Blood Cholesterol in Adults (Adult Treatment Panel III). JAMA 2001;285(19):2486-97. doi: 10.1001/jama.285.19.2486.

[23] World Health Organization. Jordan STEPS survey 2007 fact sheet. URL: https://cdn.who.int/media/docs/default-source/ncds/ncd-surveillance/data-reporting/jordan/steps/2007-fact-sheet-jordan.pdf?sfvrsn=df1a70ea_2 &download=true.

[24] World Bank. Jordan: Overview of tobacco use, tobacco control, legislation, and taxation. URL: https://openknowledge.worldbank.org/handle/10986/31954#:~: text=Jordan%20adopted%20the%20National%20tobacco,by%2030%20percent%20by%202025.

[25] Leiva AM, Petermann-Rocha F, Martínez-Sanguinetti MA, Troncoso-Pantoja C, Concha Y, Garrido-Méndez A, et al. Asociación de un índice de estilos de vida saludable con factores de riesgo cardiovascular en población chilena. [Association of a healthy lifestyle index with cardiovascular risk factors in Chileans adults]. Rev Med Chil 2018;146(12):1405-p14. doi: 10.4067/s0034-98872018001201405.

[26] Bustami M, Matalka KZ, Mallah E, Abu-Qatouseh L, Abu Dayyih W, Hussein N, et al. The prevalence of overweight and obesity among women in Jordan: A risk factor for developing chronic diseases. J Multidiscip Health 2021;14:1533-41. doi: 10.2147/JMDH.S313172.

Chapter 6

Yoga practice and non-communicable disease risk factors among middle-aged and older adults in India

Karl Peltzer*, PhD

Department of Psychology, University of the Free State, Bloemfontein, South Africa
Department of Psychology, College of Medical and Health Science, Asia University, Taichung, Taiwan

Abstract

In this chapter we assess the association between yoga practice and non-communicable disease (NCD) risk factors among middle-aged and older adults in India. Cross-sectional data (N=72,262, ≥45 years) from the "Longitudinal Ageing Study in India (LASI) Wave 1 in 2017-2018" were analysed. Logistic regression was used to evaluate associations between yoga practice levels and NCD risk factors. The prevalence of less than daily yoga practice was 4.4% and that of daily yoga practice 9.1%. Daily yoga practice was associated with better well-being (happiness, life satisfaction, spirituality, functional ability, better cognitive functioning and hand grip strength), and <daily and daily yoga practice had higher odds of insomnia symptoms than without yoga practice, but was not associated with depressive symptoms. Regarding health risk behaviours, daily yoga practice was positively associated with high physical activity and was inversely associated with current smoking and current smokeless tobacco use, and in unadjusted analysis with heavy episodic alcohol use. With higher yoga frequency, body mass index also increased. Less than daily and daily yoga practice was positively associated with physical

* **_Correspondence:_** Professor Karl Peltzer, Department of Psychology, University of the Free State, PO Box 339 (40), Bloemfontein 9300, South Africa. Email: kfpeltzer@gmail.com.

In: Non-Communicable Diseases
Editor: Joav Merrick
ISBN: 979-8-89113-514-7

pain, and daily yoga practice was positively associated with hypertension. Overall, higher yoga practice levels were positively associated with 6 of 7 well-being indicators, 3 of 4 health behaviours, as well as with 4 of 8 chronic conditions.

Introduction

According to the government of India, "Yoga components advocate certain restraints and observances, physical discipline, breath regulations, restraining the sense organs, contemplation, meditation and samadhi. These steps are believed to have a potential for improvement of physical health by enhancing circulation of oxygenated blood in the body, retraining the sense organs thereby inducing tranquillity and serenity of mind" (1).

It is estimated that in the general adult population in India 11.8% practice yoga (2). Globally, women (3,4), middle-aged (40-59 years) (2, 3, 5), those with higher socioeconomic status (3), higher education (4-6), and those residing in urban areas (6) are more likely to practice yoga.

Several studies showed that yoga practice is associated with better well-being, e.g., subjective well-being (7, 8), life satisfaction, quality of life (3), better self-rated health status (3, 5), higher spirituality (3), higher peace of mind (8), and functional ability (9). Yoga-based interventions have also been associated with improving cognitive functioning in older adults (10), and hand grip strength (11).

In terms of mental health, some research showed an association between yoga practice and improved sleep (3, 7), while some studies showed lower depression, anxiety, and stress (8), but several studies showed associations with higher levels of depressive symptoms (3), anxiety and depression (12), and mental health conditions (5). Regarding health behaviours, most studies show that yoga practice was associated with better health behaviours (3), lower smoking (3, 5), less alcohol use (7), higher non-yoga exercise (3), more physically active (13), lower body mass index (BMI) (3, 5, 7), but some studies found higher health risk behaviours, e.g., higher alcohol use (5), higher cannabis and illicit drug use (13).

In terms of chronic conditions, more mixed results were found. Some research found an association between yoga practice and lower hypertension (5, 6, 12), and other studies with higher hypertension (3), less diabetes (3), and more type 2 diabetes (2), lower COPD (12), higher asthma (3, 5), higher lung disease (4), and no association with lung conditions (3). Similarly, some research showed that yoga practice was associated with fewer bone and joint diseases (3), lower migraines, headaches (6), and less fatigue (7), but was associated with greaterr arthritis (3), more musculoskeletal problems (5), higher levels of face pain, neck pain (12), higher backache (6), and no association was found between yoga practice for joint problems (12, 14), dental pain, low back pain or headache (12), and falls or falls-related injuries (15). In a national study on yoga knowledge, attitude, and practice in India, no associations between yoga practice and NCD risk factors assessed (2). Therefore, this study aimed to determine the association between yoga practice and NCD risk factors among middle-aged and older adults in India in 2017-2018.

Our study

We analysed cross-sectional data from the "Longitudinal Ageing Study in India (LASI) Wave 1, 2017-2018" (16). Details of the sampling strategy and assessment procedures have been described in detail elsewhere (16). The study was approved by the "Indian Council of Medical Research (ICMR) Ethics Committee" and written or oral informed consent was obtained from the participants (16).

Health indicator outcome variables

Self-rated health status, "In general, would you say your health is excellent, very good, good, fair, or poor?" Responses were coded as "1 = poor, 2 = fair, 3 = good, 4 = very good and 5 = excellent" (16). Self-rated health (one item) has shown high predictive validity for mortality (17).

Life satisfaction, 5-items from the Satisfaction With Life Scale (SWLS) (18); Cronbach's alpha of the SWLS was 0.86 in this sample. The SWLS is valid and reliable and can be used with different populations and age groups (19).

Happiness was assessed with the question, "During the past week, how often did you feel happy?" Response options included "1 = rarely or never (<1 day), 2 = sometimes (1 or 2 days), 3 = often (3 or 4 days), and 4 = most or all of the time (5-7 days) in a week prior to the interview." (16). Single-item measure of happiness is valid and reliable in community surveys (20).

Cognitive functioning was measured with a series of cognitive tests (21).

Spirituality, four items from the Daily Spiritual Experience Scale (DSES) (22), e.g., "Do you think that you have a feeling of deep inner peace?" Responses ranged from 1 = never to 5 = every day in a week, and scores were summed, with higher scores indicating higher spirituality. Cronbach's alpha was 0.86.

Hand grip strength (HGS) based on a mean HGS (kg) calculated from four measurements (each hand twice) (16, 23).

Body mass index (BMI) was calculated based on height and weight measurements (16).

Functional disability was assessed with Activities of Daily Living (ADL) (6 items) and Instrumental Activities of Daily Living (IADL) (7 items) (24-26), (Cronbach alpha was 0.89 in this study).

Insomnia symptoms were measured using the Jenkins Sleep Scale (JSS-4) (27-29).

Depressive symptoms (≥4 scores) were classified based on the "Centre for Epidemiological Studies Depression Scale (CES-D-10)" (30,31). (Cronbach α was 0.79).

Physical activity was assessed with items on the frequency and time engaging in moderate or vigorous activities (16) and classified as high physical activity ">300 minutes/week moderate physical activity or ">150 min/week vigorous intensity or >300 min/week moderate + vigorous intensity; whereby time in vigorous activity is doubled") (32, 33).

Substance use included current tobacco smoking, current smokeless tobacco use and current heavy episodic alcohol use (≥5 alcoholic drinks on one occasion) (16).

Hypertension was measured and defined as "systolic blood pressure-BP ≥140 mm Hg and/or diastolic BP ≥90 mm Hg (based on the last two averaged of three BP readings) or where the participant is currently on antihypertensive medication" (34).

Other chronic conditions were sourced from the questions, "Has any health professional ever told you that you have…?": "1) diabetes or high blood sugar; 2) chronic lung disease such as asthma, chronic obstructive pulmonary disease/chronic bronchitis or other chronic lung problems; 3) arthritis or rheumatism, osteoporosis or other bone/joint diseases" (16).

Symptom-based pain was defined as "troubled by pain and required some form of medication or treatment for relief of pain" (16). Cronbach alpha for the pain measure was 0.81 in this study.

Exposure variable

Yoga practice frequency, "How often do you engage in any of the following activities like *yoga*, meditation, *asana, pranayama* or similar?" "Meditation, *asana* (postures), and *pranayama* (breath work) are all components of *yoga"* (1). Response options were "1. Every day, 2. More than once a week, 3. Once a week, 4. One to three times a month, and 5. Hardly ever or never," (16) and were trichotomized into "1 = hardly ever or never, 2 = One to three times a month, once a week, or more than once a week, and 3 = every day."

Covariates and confounders

Sociodemographic variables consisted of education, age group, sex, residential status (urban and rural areas, designated by the sampling design), receipt of health insurance, subjective socioeconomic status, food insecurity, and caste or tribe ("Do you belong to a scheduled caste, a scheduled tribe, other backward class, or none of these?") (16, 35).

Analysis

Frequencies and percentages were calculated for the sample characteristics. Logistic regression was used to assess the predictors between yoga practice level and NCD risk factors. Multivariable logistic regression models were adjusted by age group, sex, education, subjective socioeconomic status, place of residence, receipt of health insurance, and caste. Confounders were included based on previous literature review (5, 6, 8, 12, 13). $P < 0.05$ was accepted as significant. Statistical analyses were conducted using "STATA software version 15.0 (Stata Corporation, College Station, TX, USA)", taking the multi-stage sampling study design into account.

Findings

The sample included 72,262 middle-aged and older adults (≥45 years), 9.7% had food insecurity, 20.7% had health insurance, 37.2% had a low subjective socioeconomic status, and 46.7% belong to other backward classes. The prevalence of less than daily yoga practice was 4.4% and that of daily yoga practice 9.1%. The prevalence of daily yoga practice was significantly higher in men (10.3%) than in women (8.3%) ($p < 0.001$), those with 10 or more years of education (18.2%) versus no education (5.3%) ($p < 0.001$), higher subjective socioeconomic status (13.4%) versus low subjective socioeconomic status (6.7%) ($p < 0.001$), those living in urban areas (12.2%) versus those living in rural areas (7.7%) ($p < 0.001$), and among non-classified castes or tribes (13.5%) versus scheduled tribes (4.9%) ($p < 0.001$) (see Table 1).

Associations between yoga practice levels and NCD risk factors

In the multivariable model, daily yoga practice was associated with better well-being (life satisfaction: AOR: 2.60, 95% CI: 1.41-4.80, happiness: AOR: 1.06, 95% CI: 1.01-1.12, spirituality: AOR: 3.69, 95% CI: 2.86-4.75, functional ability: AOR: 0.74, 95% CI: 0.64, 0.85, hand grip strength: AOR-male: 4.53, 95% CI: 3.14-6.55, AOR-female: 2.30, 95% CI: 1.77-3.00), and better cognitive functioning: AOR:1.84, 95% CI: 1.54, 2.19).

In terms of mental health <daily and daily yoga practice had higher odds of insomnia symptoms (AOR: 1.21, 95% CI: 1.08-1.37) but yoga practice was not associated with depressive symptoms. Regarding health risk behaviours, daily yoga practice was positively associated with high physical activity (AOR: 1.29, 95% CI: 1.16-1.43) and was inversely associated with current smoking (AOR: 0.79, 95% CI: 0.68-0.91) and current smokeless tobacco use (AOR: 0.88, 95% CI: 0.78-0.98), and in unadjusted analysis with heavy episodic alcohol use. Higher yoga frequency was associated with higher BMI (AOR: 2.47, 95% CI: 1.94-3.15). Less than daily and daily yoga practice was positively associated with physical pain (AOR: 1.29, 95% CI: 1.15-1.46), and daily yoga practice was associated with hypertension (AOR: 1.15, 95% CI: 1.04-1.26) (see Table 2).

Discussion

The study found that among middle-aged and older adults in India, higher yoga practice levels were associated with six (happiness, life satisfaction, cognitive function, spirituality, functional ability and hand grip strength) of seven well-being indicators, three (high physical activity, less smoking and less smokeless tobacco use) of four health behaviours as well as with four

(BMI, insomnia symptoms, hypertension, and physical pain) of eight chronic conditions. The prevalence of yoga practice in this study (13.5%) is similar to a previous survey in the general adult population in India (11.8%) (2), and in the United States in 2012 (past 12 months use of yoga, 9.5%) (36) and 2017 (past 12 months use of yoga, TaiChi, and Qigong, 14.5%) (37), and in Germany (lifetime prevalence of yoga practice, 15.1%) (38).

Consistent with global studies (3-6), this study found that those with higher socioeconomic status, higher education, and those residing in urban areas were more likely to practice yoga. It is possible that that those with higher socioeconomic status have more time and resources to access yoga. Contrary to previous findings (2-5), this study showed that men were more likely than women to practice yoga, and we did not find a significant age difference in the prevalence of yoga practice. A previous study in India also showed a preponderance of male as opposed to female yoga users (39), but in a larger national study in India, males had an only marginally higher yoga practice prevalence than females (2). Comparing women with 10 years and more education with men with the same education in this study, the prevalence of yoga practice was with 17.5% similar to men (18.6%) in this study. So, one could argue that because men have higher education (10 or more years) (26.7%) than women (12.7%) in India, higher education is the determinant factor of yoga practice.

The association between a higher frequency of yoga practice and higher life satisfaction, happiness, spirituality, cognitive functioning, functional ability, and grip strength, found in this study, is consistent with most previous research (3, 7-11). Some evidence suggests that yoga practice may contribute to prevent age-related cognitive decline (40). In particular, yoga postures (asanas) have been reported to help in improving muscle strength (41). High-frequency yoga breathing resulted in a significant increase in hand grip strength (11). Furthermore, yoga exercises seem to improve balance and mobility in older adults (42), and yoga practice improved quality of life and mental well-being among older adults (43). Regarding mental health, contrary to some previous findings (3, 7), this study showed an association between yoga practice and insomnia symptoms. Furthermore, we did not find a significant association between yoga practice and depressive symptoms, while previous studies showed mixed results ranging from lower to higher depressive symptoms and mental health conditions (3, 5, 8, 12). It is possible that the yoga practice in this study was not specifically targeting mental distress, such as yoga before bedtime for insomnia symptoms; we found a negative or non-association.

Table 1. Sample characteristics by Yoga practice levels among middle-aged and older adults in India, 2017-2018 (N = 72,262)

Variable	Variable specification	Total	Yoga practice		
			Zero	<Daily	Daily
Control factors			**% or M (SD)**	**% or M (SD)**	**% or M (SD)**
All			86.5	4.4	9.1
Age in years	≤45-59	54.1	86.7	4.5	8.9
	60 or more	45.9	86.3	4.2	9.5
Sex	Female	58.0	87.9	3.9	8.3
	Male	42.0	84.5	5.1	10.3
Education	No schooling	49.5	91.5	3.2	5.3
	1-4 years	10.8	87.9	3.7	8.4
	5-9 years	21.1	84.0	5.4	10.6
	10 or more years	18.5	75.0	6.8	18.2
Subjective socioeconomic status	Low	37.2	89.6	3.7	6.7
	Medium	38.7	86.7	4.3	9.0
	High	24.1	80.7	5.8	13.4
Food insecurity	Yes	9.7	87.3	5.1	7.5
Has health insurance	Yes	20.7	87.8	4.2	7.9
Residential status	Rural	68.2	88.3	4.0	7.7
	Urban	31.8	82.6	5.3	12.2
Caste	None of below	24.9	80.8	5.7	13.5
	Scheduled caste	19.7	88.2	4.1	7.7
	Scheduled tribes	8.8	91.6	3.5	4.9
	Other backward class	46.7	87.7	4.0	8.3
Health indicators					
Self-rated health status	Scale (1-5)	2.77 (1.0)	2.76 (1.0)	2.82 (1.0)	2.84 (1.1)
Life satisfaction	Scale (5-35)	23.7 (7.5)	23.5 (7.5)	24.2 (6.8)	25.4 (7.0)

Variable	Variable specification	Total	Yoga practice		
			Zero	<Daily	Daily
Happiness	Scale (1-4)	2.48 (1.0)	2.47 (1.0)	2.51 (1.0)	2.62 (1.0)
Cognitive functioning	Scale (0-32)	18.7 (5.1)	18.4 (5.1)	20.1 (4.7)	20.5 (4.6)
Spirituality	Scale (4-20)	10.2 (4.7)	10.0 (4.7)	10.7 (4.3)	11.8 (4.8)
Grip strength-male	Scale	25.9 (7.4)	25.6 (7.4)	27.5 (7.8)	27.3 (7.2)
Grip strength-female	Scale	17.3 (5.2)	17.2 (5.2)	18.4 (4.9)	18.5 (4.9)
Body mass index	Scale	22.6 (4.8)	22.4 (4.8)	23.3 (4.8)	24.0 (4.9)
Functional disability (2 or more)	Yes	28.8	90.2	3.2	6.5
Insomnia symptoms	Yes	12.7	85.1	5.0	9.9
Depressive symptoms	Yes	27.6	87.0	4.8	8.2
High physical activity	Yes	55.7	86.1	4.1	9.8
Current smoking	Yes	12.2	88.4	4.7	6.9
Current smokeless tobacco use	Yes	19.8	88.5	3.8	7.7
Heavy episodic alcohol use	Yes	2.9	88.6	4.6	6.9
Diabetes	Yes	11.6	82.4	4.8	12.8
Hypertension	Yes	40.4	84.5	4.6	10.8
Chronic lung disease	Yes	6.3	88.2	3.6	8.2
Bone or joint disease	Yes	15.7	86.1	4.8	9.1
Physical pain	Yes	12.5	84.3	5.5	10.2

Table 2. Univariable and multivariable associations between Yoga practice level and non-communicable disease risk factors

Outcome variables		Yoga practice	Model 1: unadjusted odds ratio or exp (Coef.) (95% CI)	Model 2: adjusted odds ratio or exp (Coef.) (95% CI)a
Self-rated health status	Scale	None	1 Reference	1 Reference
		<Daily	1.06 (1.00, 1.13)	0.98 (0.92, 1.04)
		Daily	1.08 (1.01, 1.15)*	0.99 (0.93, 1.06)
Life satisfaction	Scale	None	1 Reference	1 Reference
		<Daily	2.09 (1.30, 3.37)**	1.03 (0.63, 1.69)
		Daily	6.73 (4.07, 11.30)***	2.60 (1.41, 4.80)**
Happiness	Scale	None	1 Reference	1 Reference
		<Daily	1.05 (0.99, 1.11)	0.97 (0.91, 1.03)
		Daily	1.16 (1.10, 12.3)***	1.06 (1.01, 1.12)*
Cognitive functioning	Scale	None	1 Reference	1 Reference
		<Daily	5.35 (3.83, 7.47)***	1.83 (1.41, 2.38)***
		Daily	7.96 (6.48, 9.78)***	1.84 (1.54, 2.19)***
Spirituality	Scale	None	1 Reference	1 Reference
		<Daily	1.99 (1.52, 2.60)***	1.50 (1.13, 2.00)**
		Daily	5.68 (4.40, 7.32)***	3.69 (2.86, 4.75)***
Grip strength-male	Scale	None	1 Reference	1 Reference
		<Daily	6.34 (3.20, 2.56)***	3.47 (1.75, 6.91)***
		Daily	5.45 (3.57, 8.31)***	4.53 (3.14, 6.55)***
Grip strength-female	Scale	None	1 Reference	1 Reference
		<Daily	3.38 (2.07, 5.50)***	2.59 (1.71, 3.90)***
		Daily	3.81 (2.90, 5.01)***	2.30 (1.77, 3.00)***
Body mass index	Scale	None	1 Reference	1 Reference
		<Daily	2.85 (1.83, 3.64)***	1.66 (1.25, 2.20)***
		Daily	1.61 (1.38, 1.85)***	2.47 (1.94, 3.15)***

Outcome variables		**Yoga practice**	**Model 1: unadjusted odds ratio or exp (Coef.) (95% CI)**	**Model 2: adjusted odds ratio or exp (Coef.) (95% CI)a**
Functional disability (2 or more)	No	None	1 Reference	1 Reference
	Yes	<Daily	0.63 (0.54, 0.73)***	0.74 (0.62, 0.88)***
		Daily	0.60 (0.54, 0.68)***	0.74 (0.64, 0.85)***
Insomnia symptoms	No	None	1 Reference	1 Reference
	Yes	<Daily	1.19 (1.02, 1.40)*	1.25 (1.06, 1.48)**
		Daily	1.12 (1.00, 1.26)*	1.21 (1.08, 1.37)**
Depressive symptoms	No	None	1 Reference	---
	Yes	<Daily	1.13 (0.97, 1.31)	
		Daily	0.84 (0.67, 1.05)	
High physical activity	No	None	1 Reference	1 Reference
	Yes	<Daily	0.86 (0.75, 1.00)	0.86 (0.73, 1.01)
		Daily	1.21 (1.09, 1.34)***	1.29 (1.16, 1.43)***
Current smoking	No	None	1 Reference	1 Reference
	Yes	<Daily	1.06 (0.90, 1.25)	1.04 (0.87, 1.26)
		Daily	0.72 (0.63, 0.82)***	0.79 (0.68, 0.91)***
Current smokeless tobacco use	No	None	1 Reference	1 Reference
	Yes	<Daily	0.83 (0.73, 0.95)***	0.84 (0.73, 0.97)*
		Daily	0.79 (0.71, 0.88)***	0.88 (0.78, 0.98)*
Heavy episodic alcohol use	No	None	1 Reference	1 Reference
	Yes	<Daily	1.02 (0.78, 1.33)	1.06 (0.80, 1.41)
		Daily	0.73 (0.55, 0.96)*	0.84 (0.62, 1.14)
Diabetes	No	None	1 Reference	1 Reference
	Yes	<Daily	1.18 (0.95, 1.48)	0.97 (0.79, 1.19)
		Daily	1.56 (1.31, 1.87)***	1.08 (0.91, 1.27)
Hypertension	No	None	1 Reference	1 Reference
	Yes	<Daily	1.10 (0.96, 1.26)	0.98 (0.86, 1.12)
		Daily	1.39 (1.26, 1.54)***	1.15 (1.04, 1.26)**

Table 2. (Continued)

Outcome variables		**Yoga practice**	**Model 1: unadjusted odds ratio or exp (Coef.) (95% CI)**	**Model 2: adjusted odds ratio or exp (Coef.) (95% CI)a**
Chronic lung disease	No	None	1 Reference	---
	Yes	<Daily	0.80 (0.61, 1.05)	
		Daily	0.87 (0.70, 1.08)	
Bone or joint disease	No	None	1 Reference	---
	Yes	<Daily	1.12 (0.95, 1.33)	
		Daily	0.99 (0.84, 1.17)	
Physical pain	No	None	1 Reference	1 Reference
	Yes	<Daily	1.34 (1.12, 1.60)**	1.36 (1.20, 1.77)***
		Daily	1.17 (1.04, 1.31)**	1.29 (1.15, 1.46)***

CI = Confidence Interval; ***$p < 0.001$;**$p < 0.01$; *$p < 0.05$; [a]Adjusted for age group, sex, education, subjective socioeconomic status, health insurance, place of residence, food insecurity and caste.

In terms of health behaviours, this study found, in agreement with several studies (3, 5, 7, 13), that yoga practice was associated with better health behaviours (less smoking tobacco, less smokeless tobacco use, high physical activity, and in unadjusted analysis with less heavy episodic alcohol use). Yoga may initiate a reduction in tobacco use by becoming more mindful of limited lung capacity, or those with a healthier lifestyle (non-tobacco use, high physical activity, non-heavy episodic alcohol, use) are more likely to self-select yoga practice (3). Clinical trials seem to show that yoga has positive effects on tobacco use (13, 44, 45). However, contrary to previous research that found an association between yoga practice and lower BMI (3, 5, 7), we found that yoga practice increased the odds of higher BMI. It is possible that people with higher BMI in India, who are mostly belonging to a higher socioeconomic stratum of society (46), are more attracted to yoga practice.

Consistent with some previous studies (2, 3, 12), this survey showed an association between yoga practice and higher prevalence of hypertension, physical pain and in unadjusted analysis diabetes. It is possible that people with these conditions choose yoga practice as a means of relief (3). Additionally, people may have used yoga to resolve physical pain and may have stopped practicing yoga when physical pain subsides and those with ongoing physical pain may have continued to practice yoga (3).

Furthermore, in agreement with some studies (3, 12, 14), this study found no association between yoga practice and chronic lung conditions and bone or joint diseases.

Study limitations include the cross-sectional design, and the assessment of some variables by self-report. Therefore, we cannot draw causal conclusions between yoga practice and health conditions. For example, people with certain health conditions, such as hypertension, may just be more likely to practice yoga and not that yoga is causing hypertension. A further limitation was that "similar to yoga" was included in the yoga practice variable, which may have led to the inclusion of non-yogic practices. The type, context, and motivation of yoga practice, and whether yoga was used for a specific medical condition and dietary behaviour, were not evaluated and should be included in future research. Future studies should examine the type of yoga practiced and for which specific health and well-being conditions it is used. The findings of this report may be used for future research and to design and implement yoga interventions in public education, training, and disease management in India.

Conclusion

The study found among middle-aged and older adults in India that almost one in ten engaged in daily yoga practice. Overall, higher yoga practice levels were positively associated with 6 (happiness, cognitive function, life satisfaction, spirituality, functional ability and hand grip strength) of seven well-being indicators, three (high physical activity, less smoking and less smokeless tobacco use) of four health behaviours as well as with 4 (BMI, insomnia symptoms, hypertension, and physical pain) of eight chronic conditions. Yoga practice seems to relate to better well-being and health behaviours but also to more mental distress and other physical conditions.

Acknowledgments

The Longitudinal Aging Study in India Project is funded by the Ministry of Health and Family Welfare, Government of India, the National Institute on Aging (R01 AG042778, R01 AG030153), and United Nations Population Fund, India.

References

[1] Ministry of AYUSH, Government of India. Yoga, 2021. URL: https://main.ayush.gov.in/ayush-systems/yoga/.

[2] Mishra AS, Sk R, Hs V, Nagarathna R, Anand A, Bhutani H, Sivapuram MS, Singh A, Nagendra HR. Knowledge, attitude, and practice of yoga in rural and urban India, KAPY 2017: A nationwide cluster sample survey. Medicines (Basel) 2020;7(2):8. doi: 10.3390/medicines7020008.

[3] Park CL, Braun T, Siegel T. Who practices yoga? A systematic review of demographic, health-related, and psychosocial factors associated with yoga practice. J Behav Med 2015;38(3):460-71. doi: 10.1007/s10865-015-9618-5.

[4] Saper RB, Eisenberg DM, Davis RB, Culpepper L, Phillips RS. Prevalence and patterns of adult yoga use in the United States: results of a national survey. Altern Ther Health Med 2004;10(2):44-9.

[5] Birdee GS, Legedza AT, Saper RB, Bertisch SM, Eisenberg DM, Phillips RS. Characteristics of yoga users: results of a national survey. J Gen Intern Med 2008;23(10):1653-8. doi: 10.1007/s11606-008-0735-5.

[6] Sibbritt D, Adams J, van der Riet P. The prevalence and characteristics of young and mid-age women who use yoga and meditation: results of a nationally

representative survey of 19,209 Australian women. Complement Ther Med 2011;19(2):71-7. doi: 10.1016/j.ctim.2010.12.009.

[7] Ross A, Friedmann E, Bevans M, Thomas S. National survey of yoga practitioners: mental and physical health benefits. Complement Ther Med 2013;21(4):313-23. doi: 10.1016/j.ctim.2013.04.001.

[8] Sahni PS, Singh K, Sharma N, Garg R. Yoga an effective strategy for self-management of stress-related problems and wellbeing during COVID19 lockdown: A cross-sectional study. PLoS One 2021;16(2):e0245214. doi: 10.1371/journal.pone.0245214.

[9] Ward L, Stebbings S, Cherkin D, Baxter GD. Yoga for functional ability, pain and psychosocial outcomes in musculoskeletal conditions: A systematic review and meta-analysis. Musculoskeletal Care 2013;11(4):203-17. doi: 10.1002/msc.1042.

[10] Hoy S, Östh J, Pascoe M, Kandola A, Hallgren M. Effects of yoga-based interventions on cognitive function in healthy older adults: A systematic review of randomized controlled trials. Complement Ther Med 2021;58:102690. doi: 10.1016/j.ctim.2021.102690.

[11] Telles S, Sharma SK, Yadav A, Singh N, Balkrishna A. Immediate changes in muscle strength and motor speed following yoga breathing. Indian J Physiol Pharmacol 2014;58(1):22-9.

[12] Bertisch SM, Wee CC, Phillips RS, McCarthy EP. Alternative mind-body therapies used by adults with medical conditions. J Psychosom Res 2009;66(6):511-9. doi: 10.1016/j.jpsychores.2008.12.003.

[13] Cramer H, Sibbritt D, Park CL, Adams J, Lauche R. Is the practice of yoga or meditation associated with a healthy lifestyle? Results of a national cross-sectional survey of 28,695 Australian women. J Psychosom Res 2017;101:104-9. doi: 10.1016/j.jpsychores.2017.07.013.

[14] Lauche R, Schumann D, Sibbritt D, Adams J, Cramer H. Associations between yoga practice and joint problems: a cross-sectional survey among 9151 Australian women. Rheumatol Int 2017;37(7):1145-8. doi: 10.1007/s00296-017-3744-z.

[15] Cramer H, Sibbritt D, Adams J, Lauche R. The association between regular yoga and meditation practice and falls and injuries: Results of a national cross-sectional survey among Australian women. Maturitas 2016;84:38-41. doi: 10.1016/j.maturitas.2015.10.010.

[16] International Institute for Population Sciences (IIPS), NPHCE, MoHFW, Harvard T. H. Chan School of Public Health (HSPH) and the University of Southern California (USC) 2020. Longitudinal Ageing Study in India (LASI) Wave 1, 2017-18. Mumbai: India Report, International Institute for Population Sciences, 2018.

[17] Schnittker J, Bacak V. The increasing predictive validity of self-rated health. PLoS One 2014;9(1):e84933. doi: 10.1371/journal.pone.0084933.

[18] Diener E, Emmons RA, Larsen RJ, Griffin S. The Satisfaction with Life Scale. J Pers Assess 1985;49(1):71-5. doi: 10.1207/s15327752jpa4901_13.

[19] Pavot W, Diener E. Review of the Satisfaction with Life Scale. In: Diener E, ed. Assessing well-being: the collected works of Ed Diener. Dordrecht: Springer, 2009;39,101-17.

[20] Abdel-Khalek AM. Measuring happiness with a single-item scale. *Soc Behav Pers* 2006;34(2):139–50. https://doi.org/10.2224/sbp.2006.34.2. 139.

[21] Lee J, Smith JP. Regional disparities in adult height, educational attainment and gender difference in late-life cognition: Findings from the Longitudinal Aging Study in India (LASI). J Econ Ageing 2014;4:26-34. doi: 10.1016/ j.jeoa.2014.02.002.

[22] Underwood LG, Teresi JA. The Daily Spiritual Experience Scale: Development, theoretical description, reliability, exploratory factor analysis, and preliminary construct validity using health-related data. Ann Behav Med 2002;24:22-33.

[23] Roberts HC, Denison HJ, Martin HJ, Patel HP, Syddall H, Cooper C, et al. A review of the measurement of grip strength in clinical and epidemiological studies: towards a standardised approach. Age Ageing 2011;40(4):423-9. doi: 10.1093/ageing/afr051.

[24] Katz S, Ford AB, Moskowitz RW, Jackson BA, Jaffe MW. Studies of illness in the aged. the index of adl: a standardized measure of biological and psychosocial function. JAMA 1963;185:914-9. doi: 10.1001/jama.1963.03060120024016.

[25] Lawton MP, Brody EM. Assessment of older people: self-maintaining and instrumental activities of daily living. Gerontologist 1969;9(3):179-86.

[26] Singh S, Multani S, Verma N. Development and validation of geriatric assessment tools: a preliminary report from Indian population. JESP 2007;3(2):103-10.

[27] Jenkins CD, Stanton BA, Niemcryk SJ, Rose RM. A scale for the estimation of sleep problems in clinical research. J Clin Epidemiol 1988;41(4):313-21. doi: 10.1016/0895-4356(88)90138-2.

[28] Cho E, Chen TY. The bidirectional relationships between effort-reward imbalance and sleep problems among older workers. Sleep Health 2020;6(3):299-305. doi: 10.1016/j.sleh.2020.01.008.

[29] Fabbri M, Beracci A, Martoni M, Meneo D, Tonetti L, Natale V. Measuring Subjective Sleep Quality: A Review. Int J Environ Res Public Health 2021;18(3):1082. doi: 10.3390/ijerph18031082.

[30] Andresen EM, Malmgren JA, Carter WB, Patrick DL. Screening for depression in well older adults: evaluation of a short form of the CES-D (Center for Epidemiologic Studies Depression Scale). Am J Prev Med 1994:77-84.

[31] Kumar S, Nakulan A, Thoppil SP, Parassery RP, Kunnukattil SS. Screening for depression among community-dwelling elders: Usefulness of the Center for Epidemiologic Studies Depression Scale. Indian J Psychol Med 2016;38(5):483-5. doi: 10.4103/0253-7176.191380.

[32] World Health Organization (WHO). WHO guidelines on physical activity and sedentary behaviour. Geneva: World Health Organization, 2020.

[33] Huffman MD, Capewell S, Ning H, Shay CM, Ford ES, Lloyd-Jones DM. Cardiovascular health behavior and health factor changes (1988-2008) and projections to 2020: results from the National Health and Nutrition Examination Surveys. Circulation 2012;125(21):2595-602. doi: 10.1161/CIRCULATIONAHA. 111.070722.

[34] Chobanian AV, Bakris GL, Black HR, Cushman WC, Green LA, Izzo Jr JL, et al. The seventh report of the joint national committee on prevention, detection,

evaluation, and treatment of high blood pressure: the JNC 7 report. JAMA 2003;289(19):2560–71.

[35] Legal Affairs. Issues of Social Justice: Scheduled Castes and Scheduled Tribes and Other Backward Classes – An unfinished national Agenda. URL: https://legalaffairs.gov.in/sites/default/files/IX.ISSUESOF%20SOCIAL%20JUSTICE%20%20SCHEDULED%20CASTES%20%20AND%20SCHEDULED%20TRIBES%20AND%20OTHER%20BACKWARD%20CLASSESAN%20UNFINISHED%20NATION.pdf.

[36] Clarke TC, Black LI, Stussman BJ, Barnes PM, Nahin RL. Trends in the use of complementary health approaches among adults: United States, 2002-2012. Natl Health Stat Report 2015;(79):1-16.

[37] Wang CC, Li K, Choudhury A, Gaylord S. Trends in Yoga, Tai Chi, and Qigong Use Among US Adults, 2002-2017. Am J Public Health 2019;109(5):755-61. doi: 10.2105/AJPH.2019.304998.

[38] Cramer H. Yoga in Deutschland - Ergebnisse einer national repräsentativen Umfrage [Yoga in Germany - Results of a Nationally Representative Survey]. Forsch Komplementmed 2015;22(5):304-10. doi: 10.1159/000439468. [German]

[39] Telles S, Sharma SK, Singh N, Balkrishna A. Characteristics of yoga practitioners, motivators, and yoga techniques of choice: A cross-sectional study. Front Public Health 2017;5:184. doi: 10.3389/fpubh.2017.00184.

[40] Villemure C, Čeko M, Cotton VA, Bushnell MC. Neuroprotective effects of yoga practice: age-, experience-, and frequency-dependent plasticity. Front Hum Neurosci 2015;9:281. doi: 10.3389/fnhum.2015.00281.

[41] Cowen VS, Adams TB. Physical and perceptual benefits of yoga asana practice: Results of a pilot study. J Bodyw Mov Ther 2005;9(3):211–9. https://doi.org/10.1016/j.jbmt.2004. 08.001.

[42] Youkhana S, Dean CM, Wolff M, Sherrington C, Tiedemann A. Yoga-based exercise improves balance and mobility in people aged 60 and over: A systematic review and meta-analysis. Age Ageing 2016;45(1):21-9. doi: 10.1093/ageing/afv175.

[43] Tulloch A, Bombell H, Dean C, Tiedemann A. Yoga-based exercise improves health-related quality of life and mental well-being in older people: A systematic review of randomised controlled trials. Age Ageing 2018;47(4):537-44. doi: 10.1093/ageing/afy044.

[44] Oikonomou MT, Arvanitis M, Sokolove RL. Mindfulness training for smoking cessation: A meta-analysis of randomized-controlled trials. J Health Psychol 2017;22(14):1841-50. doi: 10.1177/1359105316637667.

[45] Bock BC, Dunsiger SI, Rosen RK, Thind H, Jennings E, Fava JL, et al. Yoga as a complementary therapy for smoking cessation: Results from BreathEasy, a randomized cinical trial. Nicotine Tob Res 2019;21(11):1517-23. doi: 10.1093/ntr/nty212.

[46] Pengpid S, Peltzer K. Prevalence and correlates of underweight and overweight/obesity among women in India: Results from the National Family Health Survey 2015-2016. Diab Metab Syndr Obes 2019;12:647-53. doi: 10.2147/DMSO.S206855.

Chapter 7

Trends in low physical activity among adults in Bhutan: Prevalence and correlates of national cross-sectional surveys in 2007, 2014, and 2019

Supa Pengpid*, DrPH
Department of Health Education and Behavioral Sciences, Faculty of Public Health, Mahidol University, Bangkok, Thailand
Department of Public Health, Sefako Makgatho Health Sciences University, Pretoria, South Africa

Abstract

In this chapter we assess the prevalence and correlates of low physical activity (PA) in people 15 years and older in Bhutan from 2007 to 2019. Cross-sectional data were analysed from 10,411 individuals (15-74 years) who participated in the 2007, 2014 or 2019 Bhutan STEPS surveys, and had complete PA measurement. Self-reported physical activity and health markers were assessed. Overall, 11.8% had low, 16.3% moderate, and 71.8% high PA. In the adjusted logistic regression analysis, compared to participants from 2007, participants from 2014 (Adjusted Odds Ratio-AOR: 0.10, 95% Confidence Interval-CI: 0.08-0.13), and participants from 2019 (AOR: 0.09, 95% CI: 0.07-0.12), had significantly lower odds of low PA. Male sex (AOR: 0.65, 95% CI: 0.52-0.80) decreased the odds and having higher education (AOR: 1.61, 95% CI: 1.11-2.34) increased the odds of low PA. Sedentary behaviour (≥8 hours/day) (AOR: 2.50, 95% CI: 1.61-3.90), having underweight (AOR: 1.89, 95% CI: 1.17-3.04), obesity (AOR: 1.42, 95% CI: 1.14-1.77), and

* ***Correspondence:*** Professor Supa Pengpid, Department of Health Education and Behavioral Sciences, Faculty of Public Health, Mahidol University, 420/1 Ratchawithi Road, Ratchathewi, Bangkok 10400, Thailand. Email: supaprom@yahoo.com.

In: Non-Communicable Diseases
Editor: Joav Merrick
ISBN: 979-8-89113-514-7

having hypertension AOR: 1.40, 95% CI: 1.15-1.70) were positively associated with low PA. More than one in ten adults in Bhutan had inadequate PA. Factors associated with low PA included sociodemographic factors (study year 2007, female sex, higher education), sedentary behaviour, underweight, obesity and hypertension, which can be targeted in public health interventions.

Introduction

Physical inactivity (PA) has been found to increase morbidity and mortality (1, 2). In 2016, among adults, the prevalence of inadequate physical activity (PA) was 27.5% globally, which did not decrease significantly compared to the global prevalence of 2001 (28.5%) (3). There is a lack of data on national trends in PA in Bhutan, where most deaths (69%) are caused by non-communicable diseases (NCDs) (4). In countries in the region, for example, in Iran, the prevalence of inadequate PA increased from 23.1% in 2001 to 55.4% in 2016 (5), in Nepal the percentage of insufficient PA increased from 3.4% in 2013 (6) to 7.4% in 2019 (7) and in Mongolia thc proportion of low PA increased from 10.9% in 2005 to 27.2% in 2013 (8). In a trend study among adults in Mexico, the prevalence of low PA increased from 13.4% in 2006 to 19.4% in 2012 (9). In a national survey in 2014 in Bhutan, the prevalence of low PA was 6% (10).

Factors associated with low PA include health status, sociodemographic factors, and health risk behaviours. Sociodemographic risk factors for low PA include increasing age (11), female sex (12-16), those with higher education (12), and urban residence (17). Health status factors associated with low PA include low body mass index (18), obesity (19), hypertension (20, 21), diabetes (13, 17, 22), high cholesterol (23, 24), angina or coronary artery disease (22), and depressive symptoms (25). Furthermore, several health risk behaviours associated with low PA have been found, including smoking (15), heavy alcohol use (26), inadequate fruit and vegetable consumption (18, 27) and sedentary behaviour (28). This study aimed to determine the prevalence and correlates of low PA among individuals 15 years and older from national cross-sectional surveys in Bhutan in 2007, 2014 and 2019.

Our study

Secondary data from the 2007, 201, and 2019 cross-sectional STEPS surveys in Bhutan were analysed (17); the overall response rate was >93% in 2014 >96% in 2019 (29-31). "A multi-stage stratified sampling process was carried out to randomly select participants from the target population. An individual within the survey age range (25-74 years in 2007, 18-69 years in 2014, and 15-69 years in 2019) was selected in each household (29-31). The 'Research Ethics Board for Health (REBH), Bhutan' approved the study and participants provided their written informed consent (29-31).

Data collection followed the "WHO three STEPS methodology: step 1 included administration of a structured questionnaire (sociodemographics, medical history, medication use, and health risk behaviour) step 2 consisted of blood pressure and anthropometric measurements, and step 3 included biochemical tests (blood glucose and blood lipids)" (32). Height and body weight were measured with a "portable digital weighing scale (SECA 843), and a constant tension Myotape tape (SecaTMbrand)" (29-31). Of the three blood pressure readings using "Omron BP apparatus automatic blood pressure monitor" (29-31); the last two measurements were averaged (32). "Blood glucose, and total cholesterol were measured in peripheral (capillary) blood at the data collection site using dry chemical methods, biochemical analysis with a Hitachi 912 bio-analyser" (29-31).

Measures

PA was sourced from the "Global Physical Activity Questionnaire" (GPAQ) (33), and "calculated from the duration of moderate and vigorous physical activities (at work, transport and recreation) in a typical day and week." According to the GPAQ guidelines, physical activity levels were classified as 'low, moderate, and high' (33).

Sedentary behaviour was derived from a GPAQ item ("time typically spent sitting or reclining on a typical day?" (33). Responses in hours/minutes were classified as <4 hours, 4 to <8 hours and ≥8 hours/day (34).

Other health-risk behaviours included fruit/vegetable consumption (<5 servings/day), current tobacco use, and problem alcohol use (≥8 standard drinks for women and ≥15 standard drinks for men/week) (29-30, 35). Diabetes was defined as "fasting plasma glucose levels ≥126 mg/dL, and/or currently taking insulin or oral hypoglycemic drugs" (32). Hypertension defined as "systolic BP ≥140 mm Hg and/or diastolic BP ≥90 mm Hg or currently on antihypertensive medication" (36); raised total cholesterol (TC) ("fasting TC ≥190 mg/dl"); "Body mass index=BMI was calculated according to Asian criteria: underweight (<18.5 kg/m^2), normal weight (18.5-22.9 kg/m^2), overweight (23.0-24.9 kg/m^2), class I obesity (25.0-29.9 kg/m^2), and class II obesity (≥30.0 kg/m^2)" (37).

Sociodemographic data included sex, age, education, residence and employment status, a proxy of socioeconomic status (number of adult household members), and study year (29-31).

Analysis

The frequency and percent distributions were calculated to describe the characteristics of the study. Univariable and multivariable logistic regression was applied to estimate predictors of low PA. $p < 0.05$ was accepted as significant. Accounting for the complex study design, statistical analyses were conducted using "STATA software version 15.0 (Stata Corporation, College Station, TX, USA)."

Findings

The sample included 10,411 persons (15-74 years), 2,445 in 2007, 2,720 in 2014, and 5,246 in 2019. Two in five participants (39.8%) were men and 60.2% women, 57.2% had no formal education, 40.2% were employed, 36.7% lived with four or more adults in their household, and 60.5% lived in urban areas. Overall, 11.8% had low, 16.3% moderate, and 71.8% high PA. One in three study respondents (33.8%) had hypertension, 4.8% diabetes, and 21.1% high total cholesterol (see Table 1).

Physical inactivity in the different PA domains

Overall, 10.0% of participants reported neither vigorous nor moderate PA at work, 34.2% did not engage in transport related activity, and 59.3% neither engaged in vigorous nor moderate PA at leisure-time. This shows that the highest level of no PA was reported in the leisure domain.

Table 1. Sample and physical activity characteristics

Variable	Sample	Physical activity levels		
		Low	Moderate	High
	N (%)	%	%	%
All	10411	11.8	16.3	71.8
Study year				
2007	2445 (23.5)	58.3	17.7	24.0
2014	2720 (26.1)	17.7	10.5	77.6
2019	5246 (50.4)	11.4	20.0	68.6
Age (years)				
15-34	3653 (35.1)	12.6	18.0	69.3
35-49	3693 (35.5)	10.5	14.1	75.4
50-74	3065 (29.4)	11.8	15.0	73.2
Gender				
Female	6267 (60.2)	14.1	19.7	66.2
Male	4144 (39.8)	10.0	13.5	76.5
Education (in years)				
0	5953 (57.2)	10.2	11.9	77.9
1-10	2825 (27.1)	11.8	17.1	71.0
≥11	1631 (15.7)	15.3	24.1	60.6
Employment				
Non-employed	6209 (59.8)	11.5	17.5	71.0
Employed	4179 (40.2)	12.3	15.0	72.8
Household members				
0-2	4156 (40.0)	12.5	12.6	74.9
3	1418 (23.3)	10.3	18.8	70.9
4 or more	3817 (36.7)	12.1	18.0	69.9
Residence				
Rural	4117 (39.5)	10.6	15.3	74.1
Urban	6294 (60.5)	13.0	17.3	69.7
Sedentary behaviour				
<4 hours/day	8039 (78.3)	10.3	15.2	74.5
4 to <8 hours/day	1814 (17.7)	16.1	19.9	64.0
≥8 hours/day	416 (4.1)	23.1	25.7	51.2
Body mass index				
Normal	3057 (29.8)	9.7	15.1	75.2
Underweight	324 (3.2)	17.6	23.9	58.6
Overweight	1903 (18.6)	8.5	12.5	79.0
Obesity	4961 (48.4)	14.7	18.3	67.0
Inadequate fruit/vegetable intake	7969 (76.7)	12.0	17.1	70.9
Current tobacco use	2565 (24.7)	10.6	13.1	76.3
Problem drinking	823 (8.5)	11.0	13.3	75.6
High total cholesterol	2159 (21.1)	15.5	12.6	71.9
Diabetes	490 (4.8)	18.2	18.9	62.9
Hypertension	3504 (33.8)	13.7	14.6	71.7

Compared to the study year 2007, the prevalence of PA at work, transportation and leisure decreased significantly in 2014 and 2019 (p for trend <0.001). The proportion of no PA at leisure was significantly higher among women (72.2%) than among men (49.1%) ($p < 0.001$), significantly higher among older participants (50-74 years) (75.2%) compared to younger participants (15-34 years, 50.4%) ($p < 0.001$), and significantly higher among urban residents (62.0%) compared to rural residents (56.4%) ($p < 0.001$) (see Table 2).

Table 2. Physical inactivity by domains of activity

Variable	No vigorous and no moderate activity at work	No active transportation	No vigorous and no moderate activity at leisure-time
	% (95% CI)	% (95% CI)	% (95% CI)
All	10.0 (8.5-11.9)	34.2 (30.7, 37.8)	59.3 (56.2, 62.4)
Study year			
2007	66.4 (64.3, 68.5)	62.2 (60.0, 64.3)	77.9 (75.8-79.8)
2014	13.4 (11.0, 16.1)	38.1 (33.2, 43.2)	72.4 (68.1-76.2)
2019	7.6 (5.8, 10.0)	31.6 (27.0, 36.7)	51.3 (47.7-54.8)
Sex			
Female	9.8 (7.9, 12.0)	36.3 (30.6, 40.1)	72.2 (68.7, 75.9)
Male	10.3 (8.5, 12.4)	32.5 (28.7, 36.6)	49.1 (45.4, 52.7)
Age			
15-34	10.4 (8.5, 12.6)	32.8 (29.1, 36.8)	50.4 (47.1, 53.6)
35-49	9.2 (7.3, 11.5)	35.1 (31.0, 39.4)	65.8 (62.2, 69.3)
50-74	10.6 (8.6, 12.8)	36.7 (32.3, 41.4)	75.2 (70.9, 79.1)
Residence			
Rural	10.9 (8.6, 13.6)	33.3 (27.6, 39.6)	56.4 (52.0, 60.7)
Urban	9.3 (7.2, 11.9)	35.0 (31.0, 39.2)	62.0 (57.5, 66.4)

CI = Confidence interval.

Associations with low PA

In the adjusted logistic regression analysis, compared to participants from 2007, participants from 2014 (Adjusted Odds Ratio-AOR: 0.10, 95% Confidence Interval-CI: 0.08-0.13), and participants from 2019 (AOR: 0.09, 95% CI: 0.07-0.12), had significantly lower odds of low PA. Male sex (AOR: 0.65, 95% CI: 0.52-0.80) decreased the odds and having higher education (AOR: 1.61, 95% CI: 1.11-2.34) increased the odds of low PA. Sedentary behaviour (≥8 hours/day) (AOR: 2.50, 95% CI: 1.61-3.90), having underweight (AOR: 1.89, 95% CI: 1.17-3.04), obesity (AOR: 1.42, 95% CI: 1.14-1.77), and having hypertension AOR: 1.40, 95% CI: 1.15-1.70) were positively associated with low PA. In addition, in univariable analysis, high total cholesterol was positively associated with low PA (see Table 3).

Table 3. Associations between sociodemographic factors, health indicators, and physical inactivity estimated by logistic regression in Bhutan, 2007-2019

Variable	Crude Odds Ratio (95% CI)	Adjusted Odds Ratio (95% CI)
Study year		
2007	1 (Reference)	1 (Reference)
2014	0.10 (0.08, 0.12)***	0.10 (0.08, 0.13)***
2019	0.09 (0.07, 0.12)***	0.09 (0.07, 0.12)***
Age (years)		
15-34	1 (Reference)	1 (Reference)
35-49	0.80 (0.66, 0.99)*	0.80 (0.62, 1.04)
50-74	0.93 (0.76, 1.13)	0.93 (0.71, 1.23)
Gender		
Female	1 (Reference)	1 (Reference)
Male	0.67 (0.55, 0.83)***	0.65 (0.52, 0.80)***
Education (in years)		
0	1 (Reference)	1 (Reference)
1-10	1.18 (0.98, 1.42)	1.28 (1.03, 1.57)*
≥11	1.59 (1.20, 2.11)***	1.61 (1.11, 2.34)*
Employment		
Non-employed	1 (Reference)	---
Employed	1.08 (0.86, 1.36)	
Household members		
0-2	1 (Reference)	---
3	0.81 (0.61, 1.06)	
4 or more	0.97 (0.78, 1,22)	
Residence		
Rural	1 (Reference)	---
Urban	1.26 (0.92, 1.73)	
Sedentary behaviour		
<4 hours/day	1 (Reference)	1 (Reference)
4 to <8 hours/day	1.67 (1.27, 2.20)***	1.49 (1.12, 1.98)**
≥8 hours/day	2.62 (1.74, 3.96)***	2.50 (1.61, 3.90)***
Body mass index		
Normal	1 (Reference)	1 (Reference)
Underweight	1.97 (1.24, 3.14)**	1.89 (1.17, 3.04)**
Overweight	0.85 (0.65, 1.13)	0.80 (0.59, 1.07)
Obesity	1.60 (1.31, 1.95)***	1.42 (1.14, 1.77**
Inadequate fruit/vegetable intake	1.05 (0.79, 1.39)	---
Current tobacco use	0.85 (0.65, 1.11)	---
Problem drinking	0.92 (0.65, 1.29)	---
High total cholesterol	1.40 (1.05, 1.89)*	1.27 (0.91, 1.76)
Diabetes	1.67 (0.98, 2.85)	---
Hypertension	1.28 (1.07, 1.53)**	1.40 (1.15, 1.70)***

CI = Confidence Interval; ***$p < 0.001$;**$p < 0.01$; *$p < 0.05$.

Discussion

To our knowledge, this is the first investigation to evaluate the trends in prevalence and correlates of low PA among people 15 years and older in Bhutan. The study found that the proportion of low PA decreased significantly from 2007 (58.3%) to 2019 (11.4%), while in other studies, for example, in Iran, the low PA increased from 2001 (23.1%) to 2016 (55.4%) (5), in Nepal the low PA increased from 2013 (3.4%) (6) to 2019 (7.4%) (7), in Mongolia the low PA increased from 2005 (10.9%) to 2013 (27.2%) (8) and in Mexico the low PA increased from 2006 (13.4%) to 2012 (19.4%) (9). The decrease in low PA in Bhutan may be explained by the "implementation of community wide public education and awareness campaigns for physical activity, a nationwide 'Move for Health Campaign' and open-air gyms" in various parts of the country (38, 39). The prevalence of low PA found in this study appears to be comparable to a previous study in Bhutan (10), is higher than in Nepal (6), but lower than global rates (3) and in Bangladesh (11) and Iran (5).

Consistent with previous studies (12-16), we found a higher prevalence of low PA in women than in men, meaning that women should be particularly targeted in improving on PA. While some studies showed an increase in low PA with age (11), this study did not find a decline in PA with age. In line with previous findings (40), we found that low PA increased with higher education or socioeconomic status. It is possible that those with higher education are less likely to participate in PA due to less physical labour. While some studies (3, 15, 40) found some urban-rural differences in the prevalence of low PA, this study did not find such differences. However, the survey showed that the proportion of no PA at leisure was higher in urban than rural areas, which should indicate that leisure PA should be improved in urban areas in Bhutan. Consistent with previous research (41), this study also found that among the three PA domains, PA in leisure time was the lowest, highlighting the need to improve infrastructure and accessibility to sports and recreational facilities. Considering that better health can be achieved if PA is spread more evenly in the three PA domains, leisure PA can be strengthened to optimize health (40, 42).

Consistent with research in some countries (18, 19), we found an association between obesity, underweight, and low PA. While some research (15, 16, 18, 27, 28) showed an association between other health risk behaviours, such as smoking, heavy alcohol use, inadequate fruit and vegetable consumption, and sedentary behaviour, and low PA, we only found a significant positive association between sedentary behaviour and low PA in this study.

According to previous research (20, 21, 23, 24), we found an association between hypertension and, in univariable analysis, high cholesterol with low PA. While some studies (13, 22) found an association between diabetes and low PA, we did not find a significant relationship. Identified factors may be used in designing health promotion programmes on PA in Bhutan.

The study was limited due to its cross-sectional design and the measurement of some variables by self-report, including PA. Furthermore, some variables, such as mental health, which could be significantly correlated with PA were not evaluated in all three surveys and therefore were not included in this analysis.

Conclusion

We found that the proportion of low PA decreased significantly from 2007 to 2019. More than one in ten adults in Bhutan had inadequate PA. Factors associated with low PA included sociodemographic factors (study year 2007, female sex, higher education), sedentary behaviour, underweight, obesity and hypertension, which can be targeted health promotion programmes on PA in Bhutan.

Acknowledgements

This paper uses data from the 2007, 2014, and 2019 Bhutan STEPS survey, implemented by the Bhutan Ministry of Health with the support of the World Health Organization.

References

[1] World Health Organization (WHO). Reducing risks, promoting healthy life. World Health Report. Geneva: WHO, 2002.

[2] Vancampfort D, Koyanagi A, Ward PB, Rosenbaum S, Schuch FB, Mugisha J, et al. Chronic physical conditions, multimorbidity and physical activity across 46 low- and middle-income countries. Int J Behav Nutr Phys Act 2017;14(1):6. doi: 10.1186/s12966-017-0463-5.

[3] Guthold R, Stevens GA, Riley LM, Bull FC. Worldwide trends in insufficient physical activity from 2001 to 2016: a pooled analysis of 358 population-based surveys with 1.9 million participants. Lancet Glob Health 2018;6(10):e1077-86. doi: 10.1016/S2214-109X(18)30357-7.

[4] World Health Organization (WHO). Bhutan: Noncommunicable diseases (NCD) country profiles, 2018. URL: chrome-extension://efaidnbmnnnibpcajpcglclefindmkaj/viewer.html?pdfurl=https%3A%2F%2Fwww.who.int%2Fnmh%2Fcountries%2Fbtn_en.pdf%3Fua%3D1&clen=79512&chunk=true.

[5] Kamalian A, Khosravi Shadmani F, Yoosefi M, Mohajer B, Mohebi F, Naderimagham S, et al. A national and sub-national meta regression of the trend of insufficient physical activity among Iranian adults between 2001 and 2016. Sci Rep 2021;11(1):21441. doi: 10.1038/s41598-021-00252-3.

[6] Aryal KK, Mehata S, Neupane S, Vaidya A, Dhimal M, Dhakal P, et al. The Burden and Determinants of Non Communicable Diseases Risk Factors in Nepal: Findings from a Nationwide STEPS Survey. PLoS One 2015;10(8):e0134834. doi: 10.1371/journal.pone.0134834.

[7] World Health Organization (WHO). Nepal STEPS survey 2019 fact sheet. URL: file:///C:/Users/user/Downloads/STEPS_Nepal_2019_NationalFactSheet_English.pdf.

[8] Dashzeveg D, Nakamura K, Seino K, Al-Sobaihi S, Palam E. Changes in the configuration and patterns of physical activity among Mongolian adults, 2005-2013. J Rural Med 2018;13(2):151-9. doi: 10.2185/jrm.2977.

[9] Medina C, Janssen I, Campos I, Barquera S. Physical inactivity prevalence and trends among Mexican adults: Results from the National Health and Nutrition Survey (ENSANUT) 2006 and 2012. BMC Public Health 2013;13:1063. doi: 10.1186/1471-2458-13-1063.

[10] Pelzom D, Isaakidis P, Oo MM, Gurung MS, Yangchen P. Alarming prevalence and clustering of modifiable noncommunicable disease risk factors among adults in Bhutan: a nationwide cross-sectional community survey. BMC Public Health 2017;17(1):975. doi: 10.1186/s12889-017-4989-x.

[11] Moniruzzaman M, Mostafa Zaman M, Islalm MS, Ahasan HA, Kabir H, Yasmin R. Physical activity levels in Bangladeshi adults: results from STEPS survey 2010. Public Health 2016;137:131-8. doi: 10.1016/j.puhe.2016.02.028.

[12] Devamani CS, Oommen AM, Mini G K, Abraham VJ, George K. Levels of physical inactivity in rural and urban Tamil Nadu, India: A cross-sectional study. J Clin Prev Cardiol 2019;8:13-7.

[13] Sahebkar M, Heidarian Miri H, Noormohammadpour P, Akrami R, Mansournia N, Tavana B, et al. Prevalence and correlates of low physical activity in the Iranian population: National survey on non-communicable diseases in 2011. Scand J Med Sci Sports 2018;28(8):1916-24. doi: 10.1111/sms.13082.

[14] Bauman AE, Reis RS, Sallis JF, Wells JC, Loos RJ, Martin BW; Lancet Physical Activity Series Working Group. Correlates of physical activity: why are some people physically active and others not? Lancet 2012;380(9838):258-71. doi: 10.1016/S0140-6736(12)60735-1.

[15] Bennie JA, Pedisic Z, van Uffelen JG, Gale J, Banting LK, Vergeer I, Stamatakis E, Bauman AE, Biddle SJ. The descriptive epidemiology of total physical activity, muscle-strengthening exercises and sedentary behaviour among Australian adults--results from the National Nutrition and Physical Activity Survey. BMC Public Health 2016;16:73. doi: 10.1186/s12889-016-2736-3.

[16] Guthold R, Ono T, Strong KL, Chatterji S, Morabia A. Worldwide variability in physical inactivity a 51-country survey. Am J Prev Med 2008;34(6):486-94. doi: 10.1016/j.amepre.2008.02.013.

[17] Mohebi F, Mohajer B, Yoosefi M, Sheidaei A, Zokaei H, Damerchilu B, et al. Physical activity profile of the Iranian population: STEPS survey, 2016. BMC Public Health 2019;19(1):1266. doi: 10.1186/s12889-019-7592-5.

[18] Koyanagi A, Stubbs B, Smith L, Gardner B, Vancampfort D. Correlates of physical activity among community-dwelling adults aged 50 or over in six low- and middle-income countries. PLoS One 2017;12(10):e0186992. doi: 10.1371/journal.pone.0186992.

[19] World Health Organization (WHO) Overweight and obesity, 2021. URL: https://www.who.int/news-room/fact-sheets/detail/obesity-and-overweight.

[20] de Ramirez SS, Enquobahrie DA, Nyadzi G, Mjungu D, Magombo F, Ramirez M, et al. Prevalence and correlates of hypertension: a cross-sectional study among rural populations in sub-Saharan Africa. J Hum Hypertens 2010;24(12):786-95. doi: 10.1038/jhh.2010.14.

[21] Giday A, Tadesse B. Prevalence and determinants of hypertension in rural and urban areas of southern Ethiopia. Ethiop Med J 2011;49(2):139-47.

[22] Kruger J, Ham SA, Sanker S. Physical inactivity during leisure time among older adults--Behavioral Risk Factor Surveillance System, 2005. J Aging Phys Act 2008;16(3):280-91. doi: 10.1123/japa.16.3.280.

[23] Wirth K, Klenk J, Brefka S, Dallmeier D, Faehling K, Roqué I Figuls M, et al. Biomarkers associated with sedentary behaviour in older adults: A systematic review. Ageing Res Rev 2017;35:87-111. doi: 10.1016/j.arr.2016.12.002.

[24] Milton K, Macniven R, Bauman A. Review of the epidemiological evidence for physical activity and health from low- and middle-income countries. Glob Public Health 2014;9(4):369-81. doi: 10.1080/17441692.2014.894548.

[25] Ku PW, Fox KR, Chen LJ, Chou P. Physical activity and depressive symptoms in older adults: 11-year follow-up. Am J Prev Med 2012;42(4):355-62. doi: 10.1016/j.amepre.2011.11.010.

[26] Jakkaew N, Pinyopornpanish K, Jiraporncharoen W, Wisetborisut A, Jiraniramai S, Hashmi A, et al. Risk of harm from alcohol use and heavy alcohol consumption: Its association with other NCD risk factors in Thailand. Sci Rep 2019;9(1):16343. doi: 10.1038/s41598-019-52754-w.

[27] Pengpid S, Peltzer K. Prevalence, social and health correlates of physical inactivity among community-dwelling older adults in Indonesia. AJPHES 2018;24(1):27-39.

[28] Dendup T, Zhao Y, Edi Putra IGN, Dorji T, Tenzin C. Correlates of Sedentary Behavior among Bhutanese Adults: Findings from the 2014 Bhutan STEPS Survey Data. Korean J Fam Med 2021;42(4):288-96. doi: 10.4082/kjfm.20.0059.

[29] Ministry of Health 2009. Report on 2007 Steps Survey for Risk Factors and Prevalence of Noncommunicable Diseases in Thimphu. URL: https://extranet.who.int/ncdsmicrodata/index.php/catalog/738/related-materials.

[30] World Health Organization, Regional Office for South-East Asia. National survey for noncommunicable disease risk factors and mental health using WHO STEPS approach in Bhutan, 2014 URL: https://extranet.who.int/ncdsmicrodata/index.php/catalog/427/related-materials.

[31] Department of Public Health, Ministry of Health. Non-communicable disease risk factors: Bhutan STEPS survey 2019, Thimphu, 2020. URL: https://extranet.who.int/ncdsmicrodata/index.php/catalog/855/related-materials.

[32] World Health Organization (WHO). STEPwise approach to surveillance (STEPS), 2018. URL: https://www.who.int/ncds/surveillance/steps/en/.

[33] 33 Armstrong T, Bull F. Development of the World Health Organization Global Physical Activity Questionnaire (GPAQ). J Public Health 2006;14:66–70.

[34] van der Ploeg HP, Chey T, Korda RJ, Banks E, Bauman A. Sitting time and all-cause mortality risk in 222 497 Australian adults. Arch Intern Med 2012;172(6):494-500. doi: 10.1001/archinternmed.2011.2174.

[35] Centers for Disease Control and Prevention (CDC). Dietary guidelines for alcohol, 2020. URL: https://www.cdc.gov/alcohol/fact-sheets/moderate-drinking.htm

[36] Chobanian AV, Bakris GL, Black HR, Cushman WC, Green LA, Izzo JL et al. Seventh report of the Joint National Committee of Prevention, Detection, Evaluation, and Treatment of High Blood Pressure. Hypertension 2003;42(6):1206–52. http://dx.doi.org/10.1161/01.HYP.0000107251.49515.c2

[37] Wen CP, David Cheng TY, Tsai SP, Chan HT, Hsu HL, et al. Are Asians at greater mortality risks for being overweight than Caucasians? Redefining obesity for Asians. Public Health Nutr 2009;12(4):497-506. doi: 10.1017/S1368980008002802.

[38] United Nations Interagency Task Force on the Prevention and Control of Noncommunicable Diseases. Joint Mission, Bhutan, 6–10 February 2017. Geneva: World Health Organization, 2017.

[39] Tuangratananon T, Wangmo S, Widanapathirana N, Pongutta S, Viriyathorn S, Patcharanarumol W, et al. Implementation of national action plans on noncommunicable diseases, Bhutan, Cambodia, Indonesia, Philippines, Sri Lanka, Thailand and Viet Nam. Bull World Health Organ 2019;97(2):129-41. doi: 10.2471/BLT.18.220483.

[40] Pedisic Z, Shrestha N, Loprinzi PD, Mehata S, Mishra SR. Prevalence, patterns, and correlates of physical activity in Nepal: findings from a nationally representative study using the Global Physical Activity Questionnaire (GPAQ). BMC Public Health 2019;19(1):864. doi: 10.1186/s12889-019-7215-1.

[41] Strain T, Wijndaele K, Garcia L, Cowan M, Guthold R, Brage S, et al. Levels of domain-specific physical activity at work, in the household, for travel and for leisure among 327 789 adults from 104 countries. Br J Sports Med 2020;54(24):1488-97. doi: 10.1136/bjsports-2020-102601.

[42] Pedišić Ž, Dumuid D, Olds T. Integrating sleep, sedentary behaviour, and physical activity research in the emerging field of time-use epidemiology: definitions, concepts, statistical methods, theoretical framework, and future directions. Kinesiology 2017;49:252–69.

Chapter 8

Dental service utilisation in the general adult population in Eswatini: Results of a national STEPS survey

Busisiwe Ntuli[1], DrPH
and Supa Pengpid[1,2,*], DrPH
[1]Department of Public Health, Sefako Makgatho Health Sciences University, Pretoria, South Africa
[2]Department of Health Education and Behavioral Sciences, Faculty of Public Health, Mahidol University, Bangkok, Thailand

Abstract

In this chapter we estimate dental service utilization (DSU) in a community-based national survey among adults in Eswatini. National data were analyzed from 3,278 individuals (15-69 years) that took part in the Eswatini cross-sectional STEPS survey in 2014. DSU data was measured, including health/lifestyle, enabling, predisposing and need factors of DSU. Results indicate that 51.5% of participants had never DSU, 12.7% within the past 12 months and 35.8% more than 12 months ago. Predisposing factors including secondary or more education (ARRR: 4.79, 95% CI: 2.86, 8.01), enabling factors, including ever screened for glucose (ARRR: 2.14, 95% CI: 1.28, 3.56), health and lifestyle factors, including overweight/obesity (ARRR: 1.78, 95% CI: 1.19, 2.67), and teeth cleaning (≥wice/day) (ARRR: 3.85, 95% CI: 1.42, 10.47), and need factors, including pain in teeth, gum or mouth (ARRR:

* ***Correspondence:*** Professor Supa Pengpid, Department of Health Education and Behavioral Sciences, Faculty of Public Health, Mahidol University, 420/1 Ratchawithi Road, Ratchathewi, Bangkok 10400, Thailand. Email: supaprom@yahoo.com.

In: Non-Communicable Diseases
Editor: Joav Merrick
ISBN: 979-8-89113-514-7

5.20, 95% CI: 3.31, 8.19), chewing difficulty (ARRR: 2.62, 95% CI: 1.68, 4.12), and missing work because of teeth or mouth (ARRR: 2.64, 95% CI: 1.12, 6.23), were positively associated with past 12-month DSU. In addition, older age (ARRR: 2.81, 95% CI: 2.07, 3.82), and perceived poor oral health (ARRR: 1.90, 95% CI: 1.26, 2.87) were positively, and moderate physical activity (ARRR: 0.65, 95% CI: 0.43, 0.99) was negatively associated with >12-months DSU. More than one in ten participants had past 12-month DSU and several associated factors were identified. Oral health promotion needs to improve preventive DSU.

Introduction

Oral diseases are a major public health concern, including in lower resourced countries (1). Worldwide, more than 2.2 billion have dental caries and almost 10% have severe periodontal diseases (1). Other oral health conditions include oral cancers, cleft lip and palate, oro-dental trauma, noma, and oral manifestations of HIV (1). In an oral health survey in Eswatini:

> "Oral hygiene was generally poor, visible soft deposits being prevalent in all age groups and calculus in adults. Advanced periodontal disease was present in most people over 35 years of age, and intense gingivitis was widespread in all age groups. Dental caries was found to be a common problem, affecting practically every person, in many cases quite severely" (2)

Eswatini, a lower middle-income country, in Southern Africa, has a total population of 1.1 million, 88.4% are literate and life expectancy at birth is 59.1 years (3). In 2020 there were 22 dentists (0.19 per 10,000 population) and 28 dental assistants and therapists in Eswatini (4). "Most Swazis have never visited a dentist, because in a country where 70 percent of the population lives in absolute poverty, oral hygiene is considered a luxury" (5).

Among adults in communities in lower middle-income countries, 60% expressed a need for dental service utilisation (DSU) (6). Timely DSU is required for treating and preventing oral diseases, and consequently it is relevant to identify barriers and facilitating factors of DSU (7). Yet, we seem not have national data on DSU in Eswatini.

Globally, regular preventive DSU was 54% (8), and past 12-month DSU was 56% in Iran (15-64 years) (9), 13.4% in Sudan 13.4% (18-69 years) (10), and 8.3% in Solomon Islands 8.3% (18-69 years) (11). The proportion of never-DSU in adult community surveys was low in Brazil (3.3%) (12), and high in Sudan (64.6%) (10), and Nigeria (73.6%) (13). Self-reported motivation for DSU was mainly for acute treatment [54.9% in Nigeria (13); 66.9% in Sudan (10); and 74.4% in the Solomon Islands (11)] rather than routine dental check-up [24.9% in Nigeria (13), 5.0% in Sudan (10) and 5.3% in the Solomon Islands (11)].

Fcators associated with predisposing factors of DSU, as reviewed previously (10), include age, higher socioeconomic status, and female sex. Factors associated with enabling factors of DSU include urban residence, easily accessible dentist, oral health literacy and having health insurance (10). Factors associated with health and lifestyle factors of DSU include no substance use, healthy diet, being physically active, normal body weight, having chronic conditions, and good perceived health status (10). As reviewed before (10), factors associated with perceived need factors of DSU include teeth, gum or mouth problems and difficulties. The study aimed to evaluate the prevalence of DSU and its associated factors in a national community-based survey among adults in Bangladesh.

Our study

Cross-sectional data from the national "2014 Eswatini STEPS Survey" were analysed (response rate 76%) (14). Detailed methodology has been published (15). The study was approved by the "Swaziland Scientific and Ethics Committee (SEC) (Ref = MH:599)" and participants gave written informed (15).

Measures

DSU was sourced from the item, "How long has it been since you last saw a dentist?" Responses ranged from 1 = "<6 months to 8 = never received dental care" (15). In addition, respondents were questioned about the "main reason for their last visit to the dentist." (15) (see details in Table 2). Predisposing indicators consisted of education, sex, and age (15). Enabling indicators consisted of ever screened by a doctor or other health care worker for "blood pressure", and "blood sugar (diabetes)" (15).

Health and lifestyle factors

Health factors included *Body Mass Index* (BMI) calculated based on measured body height and weight, and "overweight or obesity was classified as 25+ kg/m^2" (16). Hypertension, diabetes, heart attack or stroke were assessed by self-reported health care provider diagnosis (15).

Lifestyle factors included current, past and never tobacco use ("cigarettes, hand-rolled, cigars, water pipes/shisha or pipes/kiko, snuff, chewing tobacco, kuber..pan"), heavy episodic drinking (≥1 times: "six or more standard alcoholic drinks in a single drinking occasion during the past 30 days," daily fruit and vegetable intake (15), and physical activity levels based on the "Global Physical Activity Questionnaire." (17).

Oral health-related behaviour included: "How often do you clean your teeth?" ("1 = never to 7 = twice or more a day" (15).

Need factors

Self-rated oral health was assessed with two items, 1) "How would you describe the state of your teeth and 2) How would you describe the state of your gums?" (15). Poor perceived oral health was defned as "having poor or very poor status of teeth and/or gums, and good oral health as having an average, good, very good or excellent status of teeth and/or gums" (10). Physical symptoms: "During the past 12 months, did your teeth, gums or mouth cause any pain, swelling, bleeding or discomfort?" ("Yes/No") (15). Oral health impact (OHI): in the past 12 months: "Difficulty in chewing foods," "Embarrassment about the appearance of teeth," "Days not at work because of teeth or mouth" ("Yes/No") (15).

Analysis

Multinomial logistic regression was applied to calculate factors associated with DSU (never DSU = reference category, >12-month DSU and past 12-month DSU as outcomes). $P < 0.05$ was indicative of significance. Variables found significant in univariate analysis were subsequently included in the adjusted model. Statistical methods used "STATA software version 15.0 (Stata Corporation, College Station, Texas, USA)", by considering the complex study design (multi-stage sampling and weighting) (15).

Our findings

The total sample included 3,278 adults (15-69 years, median age 27, interquartile range 20) with complete DSU measurement, 65.3% were females, and 43.4% had secondary or more education. Majority of participants (60.8%) had ever their blood pressure and 22.9% had ever their glucose measured. About half of the participants were overweight/obese (51.7%), 17.8% had hypertension, 4.1% had a history of heart attack or stroke, and 3.1% had diabetes. Most of the repondents (95.5%) cleaned their teeth at least twice a day, 4.3% were past and 7.9% current tobacco users, and 7.6% were current heavy episodic drinkers. Most participants (92.2%) ate inadequate fruit/vegetable servings, and 55.3% engaged in high physical activity. Regarding need factors, 28.9% of participants reported past 12-month "pain in teeth, gum or mouth," perceived poor oral health status (18.7%), 18.3% had difficulty chewing foods, 6.1% felt embarrassed because of their teeth, and 3.8% missed work because of their teeth or mouth. More than half of the participants (51.5%) had never DSU, 12.7% within the past 12 months and 35.8% more than 12 months ago (see Table 1).

Motivations for the most recent DSU was "pain or trouble with teeth, gums, or mouth" (65.1%), "treatment or follow-up treatment" (18.3%), and "routine check-up treatment" (8.7%) (see Table 2).

Multinomial logistic regression with DSU

In the final model, predisposing factors including secondary or more education (ARRR: 4.79, 95% CI: 2.86, 8.01), enabling factors, including ever screened for glucose (ARRR: 2.14, 95% CI: 1.28, 3.56), health and lifestyle factors, including overweight/obesity (ARRR: 1.78, 95% CI: 1.19, 2.67), and teeth cleaning (≥wice/day) (ARRR: 3.85, 95% CI: 1.42, 10.47), and need factors, including pain in teeth, gum or mouth (ARRR: 5.20, 95% CI: 3.31, 8.19), chewing difficulty (ARRR: 2.62, 95% CI: 1.68, 4.12), and missing work because of teeth or mouth (ARRR: 2.64, 95% CI: 1.12, 6.23), were positively associated with past 12-month DSU. Inadequate fruit and vegetable intake (ARRR: 0.43, 95% CI: 0.25, 0.75) was negatively associated with with past 12-month DSU. In addition, older age (ARRR: 2.81, 95% CI: 2.07, 3.82), and perceived poor oral health (ARRR: 1.90, 95% CI: 1.26, 2.87) were positively, and moderate physical activity (ARRR: 0.65, 95% CI: 0.43, 0.99) was negatively associated with >12-months DSU (see Tables 3 and 4).

Discussion

National data on Eswatini show a prevalence of 12.7% past 12-month DSU, which is similar to Sudan (13.4%) (10), higher than in Solomon Islands (8.3%) (11), but lower than globally (54%) (8), and a prevalence of 51.5% never DSU, which was lower than in Sudan (64.6%) and Nigeria (73.6%) (13), but higher than in Brazil (3.3%).

In agreement with some previous investigations (10, 11, 13), the major motivation for DSU was acute treatment and only 8.7% dental check-up. This finding shows the possible ignorance of preventive DSU and inaccessibility of dental health care. There is a great need to increase DSU, including preventive dental care in Eswatini.

Regarding predisposing factors, >12 or ≤12 months DSU increased with age and higher education, which is consistent with previous studies in terms of older age (9, 18) and higher education (8,9,18, 9). Some studies (8,9, 8, 9), found a positive association between female sex and DSU, while we only found this in the unadjusted model. With increasing age dental or oral health problems may increase explaining the association between older age and DSU (13). Moreover, people who have better education may have more knowledge and greater understanding of the relevance of DSU (7, 9).

Enabling factors of >12 months and/or ≤12 months DSU included having ever screened for glucose and in univariable analysis screened for blood pressure. The latter results was also found in the Sudan study (10). It is suggested to integrate oral health into the non-communicable diseases prevention and management of primary health care, as part of glucose or blood pressure screening in Eswatini (20, 21).

Overweigh/obesity and teeth cleaning (≥2 times/day) increased the odds of past 12-month DSU. These results are similar to the Sudan study with having overweight/obesity increasing the odds of DSU (10).

Table 1. Sample characteristics among adults (15-69 years) in Eswatini, 2014

Variable	Subcategory	Sample	Dental service utilisation		
			Never	>12 months	≤12 months
		N (%[a])	%[b]	%[b]	%[b]
All		3278	51.5	35.8	12.7
Predisposing factors					
Age group (in years)	15-24	930 (28.4)	64.4	22.4	12.2
	25-34	787 (24.0)	47.7	37.6	14.8
	35-49	838 (25.6)	37.6	48.7	13.7
	50-69	723 (22.1)	35.9	55.2	8.9
Gender	Male	1137 (34.7)	55.5	34.1	10.4
	Female	2141 (65.3)	48.2	37.4	14.5
Education	<Primary	1024 (31.3)	59.3	33.1	7.6
	Primary	830 (25.3)	56.7	33.1	10.2
	≥Secondary	1420 (43.4)	44.4	38.9	16.7
Enabling factors					
Ever screened for blood pressure	Yes	1992 (60.8)	44.5	41.4	14.1
Ever screened for glucose	Yes	752 (22.9)	32.6	51.1	16.3
Ever screened for cholesterol	Yes	71 (2.2)	14.4	59.9	25.7
Health and lifestyle factors					
Hypertension	Yes	585 (17.8)	39.5	43.1	17.5
Heart attack or stroke	Yes	133 (4.1)	38.1	39.6	22.4
Diabetes	Yes	102 (3.1)	37.5	50.8	11.7
Overweight/obesity	Yes	1589 (51.7)	41.2	43.6	15.2
Teeth cleaning	≥twice/day	3132 (95.5)	50.9	36.3	12.9
Tobacco use	Never	2878 (87.8)	52.7	34.9	12.4
	Past	140 (4.3)	36.8	48.3	14.9
	Current	260 (7.9)	45.7	40.2	14.0

Table 1. (Continued)

Variable	Subcategory	Sample	Dental service utilisation		
			Never	>12 months	≤12 months
		N (%[a])	%[b]	%[b]	%[b]
Heavy episodic drinking	Yes	246 (7.6)	49.7	36.1	14.2
Fruit/vegetables per day	<5 servings	3022 (92.2)	52.6	35.3	12.1
Physical activity	Low	819 (26.5)	44.3	41.0	14.7
	Moderate	560 (18.1)	54.3	30.3	15.4
	High	1709 (55.3)	54.7	33.6	11.7
Need factors					
Perceived poor oral health	Yes	605 (18.7)	32.7	44.0	23.3
Pain in teeth/gum/mouth	past year	948 (28.9)	33.1	36.8	30.1
OHI not work	Yes	125 (3.8)	27.2	36.0	36.8
OHI chewing	Yes	601 (18.3)	30.6	35.7	33.7
OHI embarressed	Yes	201 (6.1)	32.9	38.0	29.2

OHI = Oral Health Impact; [a]unweighted %; [b]weighted %.

Table 2. Main reason for last dental visit

Motivation for most recent dental visit	**All**	**Male**	**Female**
	%	%	%
"Consultation/advice"	7.7	7.9	7.5
"Pain or trouble with teeth, gums or mouth"	65.1	64.7	65.4
"Treatment/Follow-up treatment"	18.3	17.2	19.1
"Routine check-up treatment"	8.7	10.2	7.6
Other	0.2	0.0	0.4

Table 3. Crude relative risk ratios from multinominal logistic regression with >12-month and past 12-month dental service utilisation (DSU) (never DSU = reference category)

Variable	Subcategory	DSU	DSU
		>12 months	≤12 months
		CRRR (95% CI)	CRRR (95% CI)
Predisposing factors			
Age group (in years)	15-34	1 (Reference)	1 (Reference)
	35-69	2.95 (2.36, 3.68)***	1.44 (1.09, 1.90)***
Gender	Male	1 (Reference)	1 (Reference)
	Female	1.26 (1.02, 1.58)*	1.61 (1.18, 2.18)**
Education	<Primary	1 (Reference)	1 (Reference)
	Primary	1.05 (0.76, 1.44)	1.40 (0.89, 2.20)
	≥Secondary	1.57 (1.25, 1.96)***	2.94 (2.03, 4.24)***
Enabling factors			
Ever screened for blood pressure	Yes	1.91 (1.45, 2.50)***	1.74 (1.28, 2.35)***
Ever screened for glucose	Yes	2.73 (2.13, 3.49)***	2.37 (1.62, 3.46)***
Health and lifestyle factors			
Hypertension	Yes	1.68 (1.34, 2.10)***	1.99 (1.43, 2.76)***
Heart attack or stroke	Yes	1.52 (0.94, 2.46)	2.51 (1.50, 4.19)***
Diabetes	Yes	1.98 (1.17, 3.37)*	1.28 (0.57, 1.88)
Overweight/obesity	Yes	2.16 (1.74, 2.67)***	1.99 (1.44, 2.76)***
Teeth cleaning	≥twice/day	1.96 (1.12, 3.45)*	2.58 (1.14, 5.86)*
Tobacco use	Never	1 (Reference)	1 (Reference)
	Past	1.98 (1.22, 3.23)**	1.72 (0.92, 3.24)
	Current	1.33 (0.88, 2.02)	1.30 (0.78, 2.18)
Heavy episodic drinking	Yes	1.05 (0.72, 1.53)	1.18 (0.71, 1.96)
Fruit/vegetables per day	<5 servings	0.61 (0.40, 0.94)*	0.44 (0.27, 0.73)**

Variable	Subcategory	DSU	DSU
		>12 months	≤12 months
		CRRR (95% CI)	**CRRR (95% CI)**
Physical activity	Low	1 (Reference)	1 (Reference)
	Moderate	0.60 (0.39, 0.93)*	0.85 (0.56, 1.30)
	High	0.66 (0.51, 0.86)**	0.65 (0.45, 0.93)*
Need factors			
Perceived poor oral health	Yes	2.15 (1.55, 2.99)***	3.71 (2.49, 5.52)***
Pain in teeth/gum/mouth	past year	1.84 (1.45, 2.33)***	9.12 (6.24, 13.32)***
OHI not work	Yes	1.94 (1.08, 3.48)*	6.09 (3.32, 11.17)***
OHI chewing	Yes	1.83 (1.29, 2.59)***	7.71, 5.39, 11.03)***
OHI embarressed	Yes	1.70 (1.11, 2.61)*	4.02 (2.31, 7.01)***

ARRR = Adjusted Relative Risk Ratios; CRRR = Crude Relative Risk Ratios; OHI = Oral Health Impact; ***$p < 0.001$, ** $p < 0.01$, *$p < 0.05$.

Table 4. Adjusted relative risk ratios from multinominal logistic regression with >12-month and past 12-month dental service utilisation (DSU) (never DSU = reference category)

Variable	Subcategory	DSU >12 months ARRR (95% CI)	DSU ≤12 months ARRR (95% CI)
Predisposing factors			
Age group (in years)	15-34	1 (Reference)	1 (Reference)
	35-69	2.81 (2.07, 3.82)***	1.14 (0.77, 1.70)
Gender	Female	1 (Reference)	1 (Reference)
	Male	1.09 (0.82, 1.45)	1.28 (0.83, 1.97)
Education	<Primary	1 (Reference)	1 (Reference)
	Primary	1.62 (1.13, 2.32)**	1.92 (1.13, 3.23)*
	≥Secondary	2.73 (2.06, 3.63)***	4.79 (2.86, 8.01)***
Enabling factors			
Ever screened for blood pressure	Yes	1.03 (0.76, 1.41)	0.87 (0.58, 1.30)
Ever screened for glucose	Yes	1.60 (1.13, 2.28)**	2.14 (1.28, 3.56)**
Health and lifestyle factors			
Hypertension	Yes	0.90 (0.66, 1.24)	1.14 (0.72, 1.79)
Heart attack or stroke	Yes	1.24 (0.73, 2.09)	1.80 (0.87, 3.74)
Diabetes	Yes	0.78 (0.41, 1.49)	0.54 (0.19, 1.51)
Overweight/obesity	Yes	1.59 (1.26, 2.01)***	1.78 (1.19, 2.67)***
Teeth cleaning	≥twice/day	3.14 (1.61, 6.12)***	3.85 (1.42, 10.47)**
Tobacco use	Never	1 (Reference)	1 (Reference)
	Past	1.85 (0.94, 3.63)	1.93 (0.76, 4.94)
	Current	1.24 (0.78, 1.99)	1.43 (0.76, 2.71)
Fruit/vegetables per day	<5 servings	0.73 (0.45, 1.18)	0.43 (0.25, 0.75)**

Variable	Subcategory	DSU	DSU
		>12 months	**≤12 months**
		ARRR (95% CI)	**ARRR (95% CI)**
Physical activity	Low	1 (Reference)	1 (Reference)
	Moderate	0.65 (0.43, 0.99)*	0.73 (0.44, 1.21)
	High	0.80 (0.60, 1.06)	0.71 (0.44, 1.13)
Need factors			
Perceived poor oral health	Yes	1.90 (1.26, 2.87)**	1.71 (0.97, 2.99)
Pain in teeth/gum/mouth	past year	1.44 (1.03, 2.01)*	5.20 (3.31, 8.19)***
OHI not work	Yes	1.51 (0.73, 3.14)	2.64 (1.12, 6.23)*
OHI chewing	Yes	1.33 (0.86, 2.05)	2.62 (1.68, 4.12)***
OHI embarressed	Yes	1.46 (0.83, 2.55)	1.33 (0.69, 2.57)

ARRR = Adjusted Relative Risk Ratios; CRRR = Crude Relative Risk Ratios; OHI = Oral Health Impact; ***$p < 0.001$, ** $p < 0.01$, *$p < 0.05$.

Consistent with a previous study in Korea (22), a healthier diet (adequate fruit and vegetable intake) increased the odds of DSU. We did not find an association between higher physical activity, no tobacco use, and DSU, as this was found in some studies regarding physical activity (22) and never smoking (23).

Perceived need factors ("pain in teeth, gum or mouth" in the past 12 months, chewing difficulty, "avoid smiling because of teeth", and "felt tense because of problems with teeth or mouth") were highly associated with DSU. Similar results were found in previous research, in terms of pain in teeth or gum (10,23), chewing difficulty (10, 22), and missing work (10).

This survey identified various factors potentially influencing DSU, which has implications for public dental care policy in Eswatini. Oral health promotion strategies may specifically target populations with less or no DSU, those who have less education, those who have not screened for glucose, those not adequately cleaning teeth, those eating insufficient fruit and vegetables and who have not dental or oral health difficulties. In addition, oral health promotion needs to improve preventive DSU.

Study strength include a large nationally representative sample and the use of standardized STEPS survey methodology and assessment measures. A study limitation was that oral health and some other variables were only assessed by self-report and not clinical examination. Some potentially relevant information, e.g., on health insurance, dental care expenditure, and oral health literacy, was not assessed, and should be included in future research.

Conclusion

More than one in ten participants had past 12-month DSU and several associated factors, including higher education, ever screened for glucose, teeth cleaning (≥twice/day), adequate fruit and vegetable intake, overweight/obesity, dental pain, difficulty chewing, missing work because of teeth or mouth were identified, which can be targeted in oral health interventions. In addition, oral health promotion needs to improve preventive DSU.

Acknowledgments

This paper uses data from the 2014 Eswatini STEPS survey, implemented by the Ministry of Health with the support of the World Health Organization.

References

[1] World Health Organization. Factsheet, Oral health, 2020. URL: https://www.who.int/news-room/fact-sheets/detail/oral-health.

[2] Klausen B, Fanöe JG. An epidemiologic survey of oral health in Swaziland. Community Dent Oral Epidemiol. 1983;11(1):63-8. doi: 10.1111/j.1600-0528.1983.tb01356.x.

[3] World Factbook. Eswatini. URL: https://www.cia.gov/the-world-factbook/countries/eswatini/.

[4] World Health Organization. Dentristy personel, Eswatini. URL: https://apps.who.int/gho/data/node.main.HWF2.

[5] The New Humanitarian. Swazilands dental dilemma, 2013. URL: https://www.thenewhumanitarian.org/news/2013/04/03/swaziland-s-dental-dilemma.

[6] Hosseinpoor AR, Itani L, Petersen PE. Socio-economic inequality in oral healthcare coverage: results from the World Health Survey. J Dent Res 2012;91(3):275-81.

[7] Šiljak S, Janković J, Marinković J, Erić M, Janevic T, Janković S. Dental service utilisation among adults in a European developing country: findings from a national health survey. Int Dent J 2019;69(3):200-6. doi: 10.1111/idj.12449.

[8] Reda SM, Krois J, Reda SF, Thomson WM, Schwendicke F. The impact of demographic, health-related, and social factors on dental services utilization: Systematic review and meta-analysis. J Dent 2018;75:1-6. doi: 10.1016/j.jdent.2018.04.010.

[9] Bahramian H, Mohebbi SZ, Khami MR, Asadi-Lari M, Shamshiri AR, Hessari H. Psychosocial determinants of dental service utilization among adults: Results from a population-based survey (Urban HEART-2) in Tehran, Iran. Eur J Dent 2015;9(4):542-50. doi: 10.4103/1305-7456.172622.

[10] Pengpid S, Peltzer K. Prevalence and correlates of dental service utilisation among a national general adult population sample in Sudan. BMC Oral Health 2021;21(1):61. doi: 10.1186/s12903-021-01422-5.

[11] Pengpid S, Peltzer K. Prevalence and correlates of dental service utilization among adults in Solomon Islands. J Int Soc Prev Commun Dent 2021;11(2):166-72. doi: 10.4103/jispcd.JISPCD_400_20.

[12] Herkrath FJ, Vettore MV, Werneck GL. Utilisation of dental services by Brazilian adults in rural and urban areas: a multi-group structural equation analysis using the Andersen behavioural model. BMC Public Health 2020;20(1):953. doi: 10.1186/s12889-020-09100-x.

[13] Olusile AO, Adeniyi AA, Orebanjo O. Self-rated oral health status, oral health service utilization, and oral hygiene practices among adult Nigerians. BMC Oral Health 2014;14:140. doi: 10.1186/1472-6831-14-140.

[14] World Health Organization (WHO). STEPwise approach to surveillance (STEPS), 2018. URL: https://www.who.int/ncds/surveillance/steps/en/.

[15] Swaziland Government, Ministry of Health. WHO STEPS noncommunicable disease risk factor surveillance report, Swaziland 2014. URL: https://extranet.who.int/ncdsmicrodata/index.php/catalog/688.

[16] World Health Organization (WHO). Obesity: preventing and managing the global epidemic - Report of a WHO consultation. Geneva: WHO, 2000.

[17] Armstrong T, Bull F. Development of the World Health Organization Global Physical Activity Questionnaire (GPAQ). J Public Health 2006;14:66–70.

[18] Rezaei S, Woldemichael A, Zandian H, Homaie Rad E, Veisi N, Karami Matin B. Dental health-care service utilisation and its determinants in West Iran: A cross-sectional study. Int Dent J 2018;68(3):176-82. doi: 10.1111/idj.12346.

[19] Xu M, Cheng M, Gao X, Wu H, Ding M, Zhang C, et al. Factors associated with oral health service utilization among adults and older adults in China, 2015-2016. Commun Dent Oral Epidemiol 2020;48(1):32-41. doi: 10.1111/cdoe.12497.

[20] Biswas T, Pervin S, Tanim MIA, Niessen L, Islam A. Bangladesh policy on prevention and control of non-communicable diseases: a policy analysis. BMC Public Health 2017;17(1):582. doi: 10.1186/s12889-017-4494-2.

[21] Rawal LB, Kanda K, Biswas T, Tanim MI, Poudel P, Renzaho AMN, et al. Non-communicable disease (NCD) corners in public sector health facilities in Bangladesh: a qualitative study assessing challenges and opportunities for improving NCD services at the primary healthcare level. BMJ Open 2019;9(10):e029562. doi: 10.1136/bmjopen-2019-029562..

[22] Kim HN, Han SJ, Jun EJ, Kim JB. Factors related to oral healthcare service utilization among Korean adults aged 25-79 years. Int J Environ Res Public Health 2020;17(17):6032. doi: 10.3390/ijerph17176032.

[23] Santoso CMA, Bramantoro T, Nguyen MC, Bagoly Z, Nagy A. Factors affecting dental service utilisation in Indonesia: A population-based multilevel analysis. Int J Environ Res Public Health 2020;17(15):5282. doi: 10.3390/ijerph17155282.

Chapter 9

Enabling, disabling and need factors for cervical cancer screening among women in Bhutan in 2019

Chao Zhang[1], MD
and Karl Peltzer[2,3,*], PhD

[1]Department of Bone and Soft Tissue Tumors, Tianjin Medical University Cancer Institute and Hospital, National Clinical Research Center for Cancer,
Key Laboratory of Cancer Prevention and Therapy,
Tianjin's Clinical Research Center for Cancer, Tianjin, China
[2]Department of Psychology, University of the Free State, Bloemfontein, South Africa
[3]Department of Psychology, College of Medical and Health Science, Asia University, Taichung, Taiwan

Abstract

In this chapter we assess the enabling and need factors for cervical cancer screening (CCS) among women in Bhutan. National cross-sectional data were analysed from 2,833 women (30-65 years) who took part in the "2019 Bhutan STEPS survey". The results show that 72.7% of the women reported that they had ever undergone CCS. In adjusted logistic regression analysis, health care provider visit in the past 12 months (adjusted Odds Ratio-aOR: 1.77, 95% Confidence Interval-CI: 1.34-2.34) was positively associated, and having 11 or more years of education (aOR: 0.51, 95% CI: 0.37-0.69), current tobacco use (aOR: 0.75, 95% CI: 0.57-0.99), alcohol dependence (aOR: 0.53, 95% CI: 0.29-0.94), inadequate fruit and vegetable intake (aOR: 0.70, 95% CI: 0.50-0.98),

---

* ***Correspondence:*** Karl Peltzer, Department of Psychology, College of Medical and Health Science, Asia University, Wufeng, Taichung 41354, Taiwan.
Email: kfpeltzer@gmail.com.

In: Non-Communicable Diseases
Editor: Joav Merrick
ISBN: 979-8-89113-514-7

and anxiety symptoms (aOR: 0.41, 95% CI: 0.18-0.94) were negativelyassociated with ever having had CCS. The study showed that almost three in four women ever had CCS, and several associated factors were found that can targeted to promote CCS in Bhutan.

Introduction

Worldwide, cervical cancer ranks fourth among women (1). "Approximately 90% of deaths from cervical cancer (CC) occurred in low- and middle-income countries" (2). In Bhutan the mortality rate for CC is 7.1 per 100,000 (compared to 2.7/100,000 in the USA) (3). If CC is diagnosed at an early stage, CC can be successfully treated, highlighting the need for screening for CC (4). From 2000 the Bhutan Ministry of Health launched a national CCS programme, with CCS recommended every 3years to women aged 25–65 years (4, 5). Women who consult outpatient clinics in two hospitals for cervical cancer screening (CCS) in Thimphu, Bhutan, their previous attendance at CCS was (59%) (6). Data from 55 low- and middle-income countries (LMICs) showed that among women aged 30-49 years, the median life-time prevalence of CCS was 44% (7). We were unable to identify national population-based data on CCS and its correlates among women in Bhutan, which led to the study.

Factors associated with CCS may include enabling or disabling factors (access to health care, urban residence, higher socioeconomic status, and positive lifestyle behaviours) and need factors (such as having chronic conditions, obesity, and poor self-rated health status) (7-9). The purpose of the study was to assess the enabling, enabling and need factors for CCS among women in Bhutan. Identifying predictors of CCS may help in CCS promotion planning.

Our study

We analysed data from the cross-sectional STEPS survey in Bhutan in 2019 (response rate 96%) (10, 11). According to the STEPS survey procedures, "Socio-demographic and behavioural information was collected in Step 1) Physical measurements such as height, weight, and blood pressure were collected in Step 2) A multi-stage stratified sampling process was carried out to randomly select participants from the target population. One individual within the age range of the survey (15-69 years) was selected per household (10, 11). Since Bhutan recommends CCS for the age group 30-65 years (4,5), we restricted the sample for analysis to women aged 30-65 years in our paper. The Research Ethics Board for Health (REBH), Bhutan, approved the study, and written informed consent was obtained from all participants.

Measures

Cervical cancer screening was asked with the introduction: ”The next question asks about cervical cancer prevention. Screening tests for cervical cancer prevention can be done in different ways, including Visual Inspection with Acetic Acid/vinegar (VIA), pap smear and Human Papillomavirus (HPV) test. VIA is an inspection of the surface of the uterine cervix after acetic acid (or vinegar) has been applied to it. For both pap smear and HPV test, a doctor or nurse uses a swab to wipe from inside your vagina, take a sample and send it to a laboratory. It is even possible that you were given the swab yourself and asked to swab the inside of your vagina. The laboratory checks for abnormal cell changes if a pap smear is done, and for the HP virus if an HPV test is done.”

And the question was, “Have you ever had a test for cervical cancer, using any of these methods described above?” (“Yes, No”) (11).

Other questions for those answered with “yes” on CCS.

“When was your last (most recent) test for cervical cancer?” (Responses ranged from “1 = Less than 1 year ago” to “4 = More than 5 years ago); “What is the main reason you had your last test for cervical cancer?” “Where did you receive your last test for cervical cancer?” “What was the result of your last (most recent) test for cervical cancer?” (11).

Enabling or disabling factor questions included residence status, health care visit in the past 12 months, education, current tobacco use, fruit and vegetable intake (<5 servings/day), alcohol dependence (≥4 scores on items 4-6 of the “Alcohol Use Disorder Identification Test = AUDIT”) (12) and low physical activity was assessed with the “Global Physical Activity Questionnaire” (13).

Need factors included measured general obesity (≥25.0 kg/m^2) (14); Hypertension/raised blood pressure (BP): “systolic BP ≥140 mm Hg and/or diastolic BP ≥90 mm Hg or where the participant is currently on antihypertensive medication.” (15) History of cardiovascular diseases was assessed with the question “Have you ever had a heart attack or chest pain from heart disease (angina) or a stroke (cerebrovascular accident or incident)?" (Yes/No) (11). Depressive symptoms (scores 10 or more) and anxiety symptoms (scores 10 or more) were assessed with the Patient Health Questionnaire (PHQ-9) (16) and the General anxiety Disorder Scale (GAD-7) (17).

Analysis

Descriptive statistics were used to summarize the characteristics of the sample and the prevalence of CCS. Univariable and multivariable (including variables significant at univariable analysis) logistic regression was used to predict CCS prevalence. Missing values were excluded and $p < 0.05$ was considered significant. Taking the multi-stage sampling and weighting of the data into account, statistical analyses were conducted using STATA software version 14.0 (Stata Corporation, College Station, TX, USA).

Findings

The sample included 2,833 women 30-65 years of age. The majority of the participants lived in rural areas (62.1%). Almost two in three female respondents (60.8%) had no formal education, 13.5% were current tobacco users, 2.5% were dependent on alcohol, 87.3% consumed inadequate fruit and vegetables and 11.1% engaged in low physical activity. Almost half of the women (49.4%) had general obesity, 31.4% had hypertension, 3.4% had a history of heart attack or stroke, 2.4% had depressive symptoms and 1.4% anxiety symptoms. Almost three in four women (72.7%) reported that they had ever undergone CCS (see Table 1).

Among the women who had CCS, 67.8% had CCS within the last two years. The main reasons for the last CCS were "part of rountine check-up" (65.9%) and recommended by a health care provider (25.9%). The location of the last CCS was the Basic Health Unit I or II (46.7%), hospital (32.9%) and regional referral hospital (18.9%), and the result of the last CCS was normal/negative (86.9%), abnormal (5.5%) and suspect cancer (0.1%) (see Table 2).

Table 1. Sample characteristics of women aged 25-65 years, Bhutan 2019

Variable	Sub-category	Sample	Ever cervical cancer screening
		N (%)	N (%)
All		2833	2060 (72.7)
Enabling/disabling factors			
Residence	Rural	1819 (62.1)	1328 (74.7)
	Urban	1064 (37.9)	732 (69.40
Health care visit in the past 12 month	No	577 (20.5)	358 (63.6)
	Yes	2307 (79.5)	1702 (75.0)
Wealth index	Low	1111 (38.6)	770 (71.8)
	Medium	578 (18.9)	422 (72.2)
	High	1194 (42.5)	868 (73.7)
Education in years	No schooling	1743 (60.8)	1257 (74.2)
	1-10	709 (24.1)	539 (76.1)
	≥11	400 (15.2)	238 (60.1)
Current tobacco use	No	2491 (86.5)	1817 (73.6)
	Yes	392 (13.5)	243 (66.5)
Alcohol dependence	No	2806 (7.6)	2022 (73.0)
	Yes	77 (2.4)	38 (58.1)
Fruit and vegetable intake (<5 servings/day)	No	383 (12.7)	285 (78.2)
	Yes	2489 (87.3)	1767 (72.0)
Low physical activity	No	2400 (88.9)	1705 (72.2)
	Yes	318 (11.1)	233 (75.7)

Table 1. (Continued)

Variable	**Sub-category**	**Sample**	**Ever cervical cancer screening**
		N (%)	**N (%)**
Need factors			
General obesity	General obesity	General obesity	General obesity
Hypertension	No	1980 (68.6)	1410 (72.7)
	Yes	902 (31.4)	650 (72.9)
Heart attack or stroke	No	2790 (96.6)	1990 (72.5)
	Yes	93 (3.4)	70 (77.4)
Depressive symptoms	No	2818 (97.6)	2023 (72.9)
	Yes	65 (2.4)	37 (64.3)
Anxiety symptoms	No	2844 (98.6)	2041 (73.0)
	Yes	39 (1.4)	19 (52.5)

Table 2. Characteristics of cervical cancer screening among those who ever screened (N = 2,060)

Variable	Sub-categories	N (%)
Last cervical cancer test	<1 year ago	783 (36.1)
	1-2 years ago	627 (31.7)
	3-5 years ago	327 (16.3)
	>5 years ago	306 (15.1)
	Do not know	16 (0.7)
	Refused	1 (0.1)
Main reason for the last cervical cancer test	Part of routine check-up	1333 (65.9)
	Recommendation of the health care provider	541 (25.9)
	Experiencing pain or other symptoms	47 (2.2)
	Other	142 (6.1)
Location of last cervical cancer test	Basic Health Unit I or II	975 (46.7)
	Hospital	703 (32.9)
	Regional referral hospital	341 (18.9)
	Other	41 (1.7)
Result of the last cervical cancer test	Normal/negative	1762 (86.9)
	Abnormal/positive	133 (5.5)
	Suspect cancer	1 (0.1)
	Did not get result	142 (6.5)
	Inconclusive	3 (0.1)
	Do not know	18 (0.9)

Table 3. Associations with ever cervical cancer screening

Variable	Sub-category	UOR (95% CI)	AOR (95% CI)
Enabling/disabling factors			
Residence	Rural	1 (Reference)	---
	Urban	0.77 (0.58-1.02)	
Health care visit in the past 12 month	No	1 (Reference)	1 (Reference)
	Yes	1.73 (1.32-2.28)***	1.77 (1.34-2.34)***
Wealth index	Low	1 (Reference)	---
	Medium	1.03 (0.70-1.50)	
	High	1.12 (0.83-1.52)	
Education in years	No schooling	1 (Reference)	1 (Reference)
	1-10	1.12 (0.83-1.51)	1.05 (0.77-1.41)
	≥11	0.53 (0.39-0.72)***	0.51 (0.37-0.69)***
Current tobacco use	No	1 (Reference)	1 (Reference)
	Yes	0.72 (0.55-0.94)*	0.75 (0.57-0.99)*
Alcohol dependence	No	1 (Reference)	1 (Reference)
	Yes	0.52 (0.31-0.87)*	0.53 (0.29-0.94)*
Fruit and vegetable intake (<5 servings/day)	No	1 (Reference)	1 (Reference)
	Yes	0.70 (0.50-0.97)*	0.70 (0.50-0.98)*
Low physical activity	No	1 (Reference)	---
	Yes	1.24 (0.86-1.80)	

Variable	**Sub-category**	**UOR (95% CI)**	**AOR (95% CI)**
Need factors			
General obesity	General obesity	General obesity	General obesity
Hypertension	Hypertension	Hypertension	Hypertension
Heart attack or stroke	No	1 (Reference)	---
	Yes	1.31 (0.65-2.64)	
Depressive symptoms	No	1 (Reference)	---
	Yes	0.68 (0.33-1.37)	
Anxiety symptoms	No	1 (Reference)	1 (Reference)
	Yes	0.41 (0.18-0.98)*	0.41 (0.18-0.94)*

UOR = Unadjusted Odds Ratio; AOR = Adjusted Odds Ratio; *$p < 0.05$, **$p < 0.01$, ***$p < 0.001$.

Associations with cervical cancer screening uptake

In adjusted logistic regression analysis, health care provider visit in the past 12 months (adjusted Odds Ratio-aOR: 1.77, 95% Confidence Interval-CI: 1.34-2.34) was positively associated, and having 11 or more years of education (aOR: 0.51, 95% CI: 0.37-0.69), current tobacco use (aOR: 0.75, 95% CI: 0.57-0.99), alcohol dependence (aOR: 0.53, 95% CI: 0.29-0.94), inadequate fruit and vegetable intake (aOR: 0.70, 95% CI: 0.50-0.98), and anxiety symptoms (aOR: 0.41, 95% CI: 0.18-0.94) were negatively associated with ever having had CCS (see Table 3).

Discussion

In this national population-based survey among women in Bhutan, the prevalence of ever CCS (72.7%) was higher than in hospital out-patients in Thimphu, Bhutan (59%) (6). Data from 55 LMICs showed that among women aged 30-49 years, the median life-time prevalence of CCS was 44% (7). We found that women who had consulted health services (past 12 months) were more likely to have had CCS. It is possible that a general health care visit increases the chances of getting routine check-ups including CCS. Two in three women got CCS based on "part of routine check-up."

Contrary to some previous research (18-20), this study showed that lower socioeconomic status (lower education) increased the odds of CCS adoption. It is possible that because of the high proportion of CCS in basic health units women with no or lower education have better access CCS. This result may also be reflected in the higher uptake of CCS in rural areas (74.7%) than in urban areas (69.4%).

Unlike in a previous review (21), this study did not find an association between obesity, hypertension, and CCS. In agreement with some previous research (20,22), this study showed that the practice of other positive lifestyle behaviours (no tobacco use, no alcohol dependence, and adequate fruit and vegetable intake) increased the odds for CCS.

Furthermore, we found that women with anxiety symptoms, but not depressive symptoms, were more likely to miss CCS. This finding is in part in line with a study among women in the US, where women with anxiety and depressive symptoms had higher chances of missing CCS (23). Further analysis showed that there was no significant difference in the level of anxiety and depressive symptoms in the prevalence normal/positive or abnormal/positive CC results. A previous review showed that anxiety symptoms increased in indeterminate CC or positive results that required further testing (24).

Study limitations include that data on CCS and some other variables were assessed by self-report, and the cross-sectional study design. Future studies should include questions on knowledge and attitudes about cancer and CCS.

Conclusion

The study showed that in this national survey almost three in four women ever had CCS in Bhutan. Several factors associated with non-CSS, including non-health care provider visit (past 12 months), higher education, current tobacco use, alcohol dependence, inadequate fruit and vegetable intake, and anxiety symptoms, can be included in targeted interventions.

Acknowledgments

This paper uses data from the 2019 Bhutan STEPS survey, implemented by the Bhutan Ministry of Health with the support of the World Health Organization.

References

[1] World Health Organization. Cervical cancer, 2022. URL: https://www.who.int/news-room/fact-sheets/detail/cervical-cancer.

[2] Sung H, Ferlay J, Siegel RL, Laversanne M, Soerjomataram I, Jemal A, et al. Global cancer statistics 2020: GLOBOCAN estimates of incidence and mortality worldwide for 36 cancers in 185 countries. CA Cancer J Clin 2021:71:209–49. doi:10.3322/caac.21660.

[3] Ferlay J, Soerjomataram I, Ervik M, Dikshit R, Eser S, Mathers C, et al. GLOBOCAN 2012 v1.0, Cancer incidence and mortality worldwide: IARC Cancer Base No. 11. http://globocan.iarc.fr/Pages/fact_sheets_population.aspx.

[4] Ministry of Health, Bhutan. Cervical cancer screening manual, 2014. URL: https://www.moh.gov.bt/wp-content/uploads/ict-files/2014/11/Cervical-Cancer-screening-manual-2014.pdf.

[5] Baussano I, Tshering S, Choden T, Lazzarato F, Tenet V, Plummer M, et al. Cervical cancer screening in rural Bhutan with the careHPV test on self-collected samples: an ongoing cross-sectional, population-based study (REACH-Bhutan). BMJ Open 2017;7(7):e016309. doi: 10.1136/bmjopen-2017-016309.
[6] Baussano I, Tshomo U, Clifford GM, Tenet V, Tshokey T, Franceschi S. Cervical cancer screening program in Thimphu, Bhutan: population coverage and characteristics associated with screening attendance. BMC Womens Health 2014;14:147. doi: 10.1186/s12905-014-0147-0.
[7] Lemp JM, De Neve JW, Bussmann H, Chen S, Manne-Goehler J, Theilmann M, et al. Lifetime prevalence of cervical cancer screening in 55 low- and middle-income countries. JAMA 2020;324(15):1532-42. doi: 10.1001/jama.2020.16244.
[8] Pengpid S, Peltzer K. Prevalence and risk factors for cervical and breast cancer screening among women in the general population in Indonesia. Gend Behav 2018;16(3):11994-003.
[9] Phaswana-Mafuya N, Peltzer K. Breast and cervical cancer screening prevalence and associated factors among women in the South African general population. Asian Pac J Cancer Prev 2018;19(6):1465-70. doi: 10.22034/APJCP.2018.19.6.1465.
[10] World Health Organization. STEPwise approach to surveillance (STEPS), 2018. URL: https://www.who.int/ncds/surveillance/steps/en/.
[11] Department of Public Health, Ministry of Health. Non-communicable disease risk factors: Bhutan STEPS survey 2019, Thimphu. URL: https://extranet.who.int/ncdsmicrodata/index.php/catalog/855/related-materials.
[12] Pengpid S, Peltzer K. Depression and generalised anxiety and associated factors among adults in Bhutan: Results of national cross-sectional survey in 2019. Asian J Psychiatr 2022;67:102959. doi: 10.1016/j.ajp.2021.102959.
[13] Armstrong T, Bull F. Development of the World Health Organization Global Physical Activity Questionnaire (GPAQ). J Public Health 2006;14:66–70.
[14] Wen CP, David Cheng TY, Tsai SP, Chan HT, Hsu HL, Hsu CC, et al. Are Asians at greater mortality risks for being overweight than Caucasians? Redefining obesity for Asians. Public Health Nutr 2009;12(4):497–506. https://doi.org/10.1017/S1368980008002802.
[15] Chobanian AV, Bakris GL, Black HR, Cushman WC, Green LA, Izzo JL et al. Seventh report of the Joint National Committee of Prevention, Detection, Evaluation, and Treatment of High Blood Pressure. Hypertension 2003;42(6):1206–52. http://dx.doi.org/10.1161/01.HYP.0000107251.49515.c2.
[16] Kroenke K, Spitzer RL, Williams JB. The PHQ-9: validity of a brief depression severity measure. J Gen Intern Med 2001;16(9):606-13. doi: 10.1046/j.1525-1497.2001.016009606.x.
[17] Spitzer RL, Kroenke K, Williams JB, Löwe B. A brief measure for assessing generalized anxiety disorder: the GAD-7. Arch Intern Med 2006;166(10):1092-7. doi: 10.1001/archinte.166.10.1092.
[18] Ampofo AG, Adumatta AD, Owusu E, Awuviry-Newton K. A cross-sectional study of barriers to cervical cancer screening uptake in Ghana: An application of the health belief model. PLoS One 2020;15(4):e0231459. doi: 10.1371/journal.pone.0231459.

[19] Islam RM, Billah B, Hossain MN, Oldroyd J. Barriers to cervical cancer and breast cancer screening uptake in low-income and middle-income countries: A systematic review. Asian Pac J Cancer Prev 2017;18(7):1751-63. doi: 10.22034/APJCP.2017.18.7.1751.

[20] Sözmen K, Unal B, Sakarya S, Dinc G, Yardim N, Keskinkilic B, et al. Determinants of breast and cervical cancer screening uptake among women in Turkey. Asia Pac J Public Health 2016;28(6):528-38. doi: 10.1177/1010539516654541.

[21] Maruthur NM, Bolen SD, Brancati FL, Clark JM. The association of obesity and cervical cancer screening: a systematic review and meta-analysis. Obesity (Silver Spring) 2009;17(2):375-81. doi: 10.1038/oby.2008.480.

[22] Theme Filha MM, Leal MD, Oliveira EF, Esteves-Pereira AP, Gama SG. Regional and social inequalities in the performance of Pap test and screening mammography and their correlation with lifestyle: Brazilian national health survey, 2013. Int J Equity Health 2016;15(1):136. doi: 10.1186/s12939-016-0430-9.

[23] Zhang X, Mkuu R, Samman E, Cummings S, Sherman L, Wigfall LT, et al. Anxiety and depressive symptoms and missing breast cancer and cervical screening: results from Brazos valley community health survey. Psychol Health Med 2020;25(4):402-9. doi: 10.1080/13548506.2019.1668031.

[24] Kim A, Chung KC, Keir C, Patrick DL. Patient-reported outcomes associated with cancer screening: a systematic review. BMC Cancer 2022;22(1):223. doi: 10.1186/s12885-022-09261-5.

Chapter 10

High prevalence of dyslipidemia and associated factors among adults in a national survey in Myanmar

Supa Pengpid[*], **DrPH**
Department of Health Education and Behavioral Sciences, Faculty of Public Health, Mahidol University, Bangkok, Thailand
Department of Public Health, Sefako Makgatho Health Sciences University, Pretoria, South Africa

Abstract

This chapter assess the prevalence and correlates of dyslipidemia among adults in Myanmar. In the 2014 Myanmar cross-sectional STEPS survey, 7,058 participants had complete lipid measurements. Results indicate a prevalence of dyslipidemia of 69.7%. Among those with dyslipidemia, 115 (1.2%) were aware. In both sexes, older age (40-64 years) (AOR: 1.65, 95% CI: 1.35-2.00), compared to less than the fourth standard of education, eighth standard or more education (AOR: 1.52, 95% CI: 1.14-2.03), overweight (AOR: 3.39, 95% CI: 2.28-5.03), obesity class I (AOR: 2.93, 95% CI: 2.42-3.55), obesity class II (AOR: 2.48, 95% CI: 1.29-4.78), and current smoking (AOR: 1.41, 95% CI: 1.09-1.82) were positively associated with prevalence of dyslipidaemia. Male sex (AOR: 0.61, 95% CI: 0.50-0.74), having a general body underweight (AOR: 0.65, 95% CI: 0.50-0.84) and less than daily alcohol use (AOR: 0.74, 95% CI: 0.55-1.00) were negatively associated with dyslipidemia. In gender stratified analysis, only among women and not men,

---

[*] ***Correspondence:*** Professor Supa Pengpid, Department of Health Education and Behavioral Sciences, Faculty of Public Health, Mahidol University, 420/1 Ratchawithi Road, Ratchathewi, Bangkok 10400, Thailand. Email: supaprom@yahoo.com.

In: Non-Communicable Diseases
Editor: Joav Merrick
ISBN: 979-8-89113-514-7

hypertension, and diabetes were positively associated with the prevalence of dyslipidemia. Seven out of ten adults in Myanmar had dyslipidemia, calling for public health interventions.

Introduction

Dyslipidemia is defined as "one or a combination of low high-density lipoprotein cholesterol (HDL-C), elevated triglyceride (TG), high low-density lipoprotein cholesterol (LDL-C), and elevated total cholesterol (TC)" (1, 2), has increased globally (1) and is involved in major clinical conditions, such as cardiovascular disease (CVD) (1). CVDs contribute to 25% of mortality in Myanmar in 2018 (3). In a household survey (N = 600, ≥40 years) in four townships in Myanmar, the prevalence of angina was 9%, and "possible heart attack, stroke and heart failure was 7.5, 1.5 and 2.8%" (4). Myanmar lacks national data on dyslipidemia, which led to the study. In 2013 and 2014 in a STEPS survey in the Yangon Region in Myanmar (25-74 years), the prevalence of "high TC (≥5.17 mmol/L) was 46.8%, high TG (≥2.0 mmol/L) 19.3%, low HDL (<1.03 mmol/L in men and <1.28 mmol/L in women) 53.4% and high LDL (≥4.23 mmol/L) 14.2%" (5). For example, in China (>18 years), the "prevalence of dyslipidemia was 34.0%, and 31.0% were aware, 19.5% in treatment and 8.9% were controlled" (6).

As previously reviewed (7), risk factors for dyslipidemia prevalence include sociodemographic factors (male sex, urban residence, and ethnicity), chronic conditions (obesity, CVD, hypertension, and diabetes), and health behaviour risk factors (smoking, and physical inactivity. Factors associated with awareness of dyslipidemia diagnosis include sociodemographic factors (older age, urban residence, higher education), chronic conditions (higher BMI, CVD, hypertension, and diabetes) (7). The aim of the study was to assess the prevalence and correlates of dyslipidemia among adults in Myanmar.

Our study

National cross-sectional data from the 2014 Myanmar STEPS survey with complete lipid measurements (8) were analysed; the study response rate was 90% (9). Following STEPS survey procedures:

> "Socio-demographic and behavioural information was collected in Step 1. Physical measurements such as height, weight, and blood pressure were collected in Step 2. Biochemical measurements were collected to assess blood glucose and cholesterol levels in Step 3. A multi-stage stratified sampling process was carried out to randomly select participants from the target population. One individual within the age range of the survey (18-69 years) was selected per household. Ethics approval was provided by the Ethics Review Committee of the Department of Medical Research [no approval #], and informed consent was obtained from all participants by written or finger impressions" (8-10).

Ethics approval was provided by the Ethics Review Committee of the Department of Medical Research, and participants provided their written informed consent.

Measures

Dyslipidemia was classified (11) as:

> "being on antilipidemic medication or having one or more of the following: elevated total cholesterol (TC): ≥5.17 mmol/l (200 mg/dl), high triglycerides (TG): ≥1.70 mmol/l (150 mg/dl), low HDL-C: female ≤1.29 mmol/l; ≤male 1.03 (<50 mg/dl in women, <40 mg/dl in men) and high LDL-C: ≥3.36 mmol/l (130 mg/dl)."

The awareness rate of dyslipidemia was defined as:

> "having been diagnosed by a health care provider as having high cholesterol among those with dyslipidaemia. The rate of dyslipidaemia treatment was defined as the self-reported use of lipid lowering drugs in the past 2 weeks among participants who were aware of dyslipidaemia" (11).

Central obesity ("waist circumference ≥90 cm in men, ≥80 cm in women") (12); measured *body mass index* (BMI) (kg/m^2): "normal weight 18.5-22.9 kg/m^2, underweight <18.5 kg/m^2, overweight 23.0-24.9 kg/m^2, obesity class I 25.0 kg/m^2 -29.9 kg/m^2, and obesity class II ≥30.0 kg/m^2" (13), *Hypertension/raised blood pressure* (BP): "systolic BP ≥140 mm Hg and/or diastolic BP ≥ 90 mm Hg or where the participant is currently on antihypertensive medication." (14). *Diabetes:* "fasting plasma glucose levels >=7.0 mmol/L (≥126 mg/dl); or using insulin or oral hypoglycaemic drugs." (10). Self-reported *CVDs*, "Have you ever had a heart attack or chest pain from heart disease (angina) or a stroke (cerebrovascular accident or incident)? (Yes, No)" (9).

Current tobacco use, alcohol use, and low, moderate, and high physical activity according to the "Global Physical Activity Questionnaire" (15). Sociodemographic variables included age (years), sex (male, female), education, and ethnic group (9).

Analysis

All statistical analyses were conducted with "STATA software version 14.0 (Stata Corporation, College Station, TX, USA)," taking the complex study design into account. Frequencies and percentages were calculated to describe the sample. Logistic regressions were used to estimate the predictors of dyslipidemia and its components. P-values <0.05 were considered significant.

Findings

The sample consisted of 7,058 people (24-64 years, M = 45.3 years, SD = 10.7 years) who had complete lipid measurements. The prevalence of dyslipidemia was 69.7%, 26.8% high TC, 31.7% high TG, 48.4% low HDL-C, and 22.8% high LDL-C. Among the eight ethnic groups in Myanmar, Chin (95.3%) had the highest prevalence and Shan (66.6%) had the lowest prevalence of dyslipidemia (see Table 1).

Distribution of awareness, and treatment of dyslipidemia

Among those with dyslipidemia, 115 (1.2%) were aware, and among those who knew (N = 115), 11 (6.2%) were treated.

Table 1. Sample description and prevalence of dyslipidemia and its subtypes, Myanmar, 2014

Variable	Subcategory	Sample	High TC	High TG	Low HDL-C	High LDL-C	Dyslipidemia
		N (%[a])	%[b]	%[b]	%[b]	%[b]	%[b]
Total		7058	26.8	31.7	48.4	22.8	69.7
Age (years)	25-34	1360 (19.3)	15.0	24.0	45.2	13.4	62.9
	35-44	1916 (27.1)	26.0	33.1	50.0	21.4	70.7
	45-54	2054 (29.1)	35.0	37.8	51.3	30.1	74.4
	55-64	1728 (24.5)	39.3	35.7	47.9	32.8	74.7
Gender	Female	4688 (66.4)	31.6	30.0	57.0	26.1	76.0
	Male	2370 (33.6)	21.9	33.5	39.6	19.4	63.4
Education	No schooling	1055 (15.0)	20.9	31.5	47.9	16.2	65.2
	<4th Standard	1597 (22.7)	27.0	27.1	47.7	22.3	67.8
	4-7th Standard	2612 (37.1)	26.7	29.4	49.9	23.0	69.4
	≥8th Standard	1773 (25.2)	29.3	37.6	46.9	25.6	73.3
Ethnic group	Bamar	4984 (70.6)	26.7	28.2	48.1	24.1	68.2
	Kachin	37 (0.5)	12.9	66.4	46.3	10.7	87.0
	Kayah	51 (0.7)	10.2	50.5	46.5	5.8	68.4
	Kayin	300 (4.3)	43.6	30.0	47.3	37.8	77.0
	Chin	49 (0.7)	28.0	19.2	76.2	24.5	95.3
	Mon	184 (2.6)	39.9	47.9	54.7	26.5	84.1
	Yakhine	515 (7.3)	21.4	28.5	52.5	14.8	70.1
	Shan	447 (6.3)	21.8	35.2	45.8	17.5	66.6
	Other	487 (6.9)	33.5	45.5	47.0	23.8	73.0
Body Mass Index	Normal	2807 (40.3)	21.0	23.0	40.3	18.6	61.0
	Underweight	1147 (16.5)	17.3	15.0	33.7	13.8	52.2
	Overweight	1053 (15.1)	31.9	49.0	63.1	26.7	85.6
	Obesity class I	1487 (21.3)	39.0	44.2	63.0	33.7	84.9
	Obesity class II	478 (6.9)	34.8	45.4	65.2	27.7	84.3

Table 1. (Continued)

Variable	Subcategory	Sample	High TC	High TG	Low HDL-C	High LDL-C	Dyslipidemia
		N (%[a])	%[b]	%[b]	%[b]	%[b]	%[b]
Central obesity	No	4558 (65.4)	21.5	25.6	42.4	19.0	63.6
	Yes	2414 (34.6)	38.6	44.9	64.3	31.6	85.0
Hypertension	No	4839 (68.9)	23.6	27.3	45.9	20.4	66.1
	Yes	2181 (31.1)	35.6	42.9	55.3	29.1	79.4
Diabetes	No	6531 (92.6)	25.9	29.9	47.3	22.1	68.9
	Yes	524 (7.4)	40.2	58.4	64.6	32.0	81.8
Cardiovascular disease	No	6335 (89.9)	26.4	31.4	47.9	22.4	69.2
	Yes	719 (10.2)	32.7	36.3	54.7	28.3	77.1
Physical activity	Low	1305 (18.6)	31.9	39.6	51.2	25.5	74.3
	Moderate	1536 (21.9)	30.5	32.7	50.5	25.6	72.5
	High	4182 (59.5)	24.4	29.1	47.0	21.3	67.6
Current smoking	No	5470 (77.5	28.6	30.6	50.5	24.2	71.0
	Yes	1586 (22.5)	21.7	34.7	42.4	18.8	66.3
Alcohol use	No	5916 (84.1)	28.5	30.3	53.6	24.7	72.8
	<daily	823 (11.7)	20.7	35.0	36.5	18.1	62.5
	daily	299 (4.2)	27.6	38.3	25.1	16.1	58.2

[a]unweighted; [b]weighted.

Table 2. Associations with prevalence of dyslipidemia

Variable	Subcategory	Male	Female	Both sexes
		AOR (95% CI)	AOR (95% CI)	AOR (95% CI)
Age (years)	25-39	1 (Reference)	1 (Reference)	(Reference)
	40-64	1.79 (1.31, 2.45)***	1.44 (1.17, 177)***	1.65 (1.35, 2.00)***
Gender	Female			1 (Reference)
	Male			0.61 (0.50, 0.74)***
Education	<4th Standard	1 (Reference)	1 (Reference)	1 (Reference)
	4-7th Standard	1.28 (0.87, 1.89)	1.23 (0.92, 1.66)	1.23 (1.00, 1.52)
	≥8th Standard	2.08 (1.43, 3.02)***	1.04 (0.78, 1.38)	1.52 (1.14, 2.03)**
Body Mass Index	Normal	1 (Reference)	1 (Reference)	1 (Reference)
	Underweight	0.62 (0.45, 0.84)**	0.64 (0.43, 0.95)*	0.65 (0.50, 0.84)**
	Overweight	5.38 (3.03, 9.55)***	2.17 (1.29, 3.64)**	3.39 (2.28, 5.03)***
	Obesity class I	3.34 (1.88, 5.93)***	2.57 (2.07, 3.17)***	2.93 (2.42, 3.55)***
	Obesity class II	3.03 (1.13, 8.17)*	2.17 (0.96, 4.90)	2.48 (1.29, 4.78)**
Hypertension	No	1 (Reference)	1 (Reference)	1 (Reference)
	Yes	1.09 (0.80, 1.48)	1.60 (1.14, 2.25)**	1.28 (1.00, 1.64)
Diabetes	No	1 (Reference)	1 (Reference)	1 (Reference)
	Yes	0.78 (0.50, 1.23)	1.90 (1.27, 2.86)**	1.19 (0.86, 1.67)
Cardiovascular disease	No	1 (Reference)	1 (Reference)	1 (Reference)
	Yes	1.18 (0.74, 1.88)	1.10 (0.70, 1.71)	1.12 (0.78, 1.60)
Physical inactivity	No	1 (Reference)	1 (Reference)	1 (Reference)
	Yes	0.95 (0.58, 1.55)	0.90 (0.66, 1.23)	0.93 (0.65, 1.32)
Current smoking use	No	1 (Reference)	1 (Reference)	1 (Reference)
	Yes	1.27 (0.89, 1.80)	2.76 (2.03, 3.74)***	1.41 (1.09, 1.82)*
Alcohol use	No	1 (Reference)	1 (Reference)	1 (Reference)
	<daily	0.79 (0.56, 1.12)	0.61 (0.39, 0.95)*	0.74 (0.55, 1.00)*
	daily	0.80 (0.48, 1.36)	0.71 (0.30, 1.69)	0.73 (0.45, 1.18)

***$p < 0.001$; **$p < 0.01$; *$p < 0.05$; COR = Crude Odds Ratio; AOR = Adjusted Odds Ratio; Confidence Interval.

Associations with dyslipidemia prevalence

In the multivariable model, in both sexes, older age (40-64 years) (AOR: 1.65, 95% CI: 1.35-2.00), compared to less than the fourth standard of education, eighth standard or more education (AOR: 1.52, 95% CI: 1.14-2.03), overweight (AOR: 3.39, 95% CI: 2.28-5.03), obesity class I (AOR: 2.93, 95% CI: 2.42-3.55), obesity class II (AOR: 2.48, 95% CI: 1.29-4.78), and current smoking (AOR: 1.41, 95% CI: 1.09-1.82) were positively associated with prevalence of dyslipidemia. Male sex (AOR: 0.61, 95% CI: 0.50-0.74), having a general body underweight (AOR: 0.65, 95% CI: 0.50-0.84) and less than daily alcohol use (AOR: 0.74, 95% CI: 0.55-1.00) were negatively associated with dyslipidemia. In the gender stratified analysis, hypertension and diabetes were positively associated with the prevalence of dyslipidemia only among women and not men (see Table 2).

Discussion

The national proportion of dyslipidemia in Myanmar (69.7%) was higher than in China (>18 years, 34.0%) (6), and lower than in Pakistan (≥20 years, 96%) (10). Low HDL-C (48.4%) had the highest rate, followed by high TG (31.7%), high TC (26.8%), and high LDL-C (22.8%). A similar distribution was found in the 2013/2014 STEPS survey in the Yangon Region in Myanmar (5), Pakistan (16), and China (6). High rates of low HDL-C are a risk factor for coronary heart disease (11).

Consistent with previous research (2,6,16), obesity, hypertension, older age, diabetes and current smoking increased the odds and underweight and less than daily alcohol use decreased the odds of dyslipidaemia in both sexes and/or in women. A nutritional transition in Myanmar (17) may have led to a high prevalence of overweight/obesity (43.3%) found, increasing the risk of dyslipidemia. Tobacco use is a known risk factor to impair insulin and may be implicated in insulin resistance (18). Unlike some previous research that showed that physical activity was protective against dyslipidemia (2), we did not find this association.

We found that female sex was associated with dyslipidemia, unlike some studies in China (6, 19). Furthermore, we found that the prevalence of dyslipidemia was the highest among Chin (95.3%) and the lowest among Shan (66.6%), demonstrating the importance of ethnic differences, which should be considered in intervention strategies (20). The proportion of dyslipidemia awareness (1.2%), and treatment (6.2%), was much lower than for example in China (awareness: 31.0% and treatment: 19.5%) (6), calling for increased efforts of opportunistic screening in Myanmar.

Study limitations include the cross-sectional study design and some data were assessed by self-report. Future studies may include additional measures, such as a family history of hyperlipidemia and dietary behaviour.

Conclusion

In Myanmar, a high rate of dyslipidemia was found, calling for improved public health interventions, including screening, better diagnosis, treatment, and control of dyslipidemia.

Acknowledgment

This paper uses data from the 2014 Myanmar STEPS survey, implemented by the National Institute of Preventive and Social Medicine with the support of the World Health Organization.

References

[1] Pirillo A, Casula M, Olmastroni E, Norata GD, Catapano AL. Global epidemiology of dyslipidaemias. Nat Rev Cardiol 2021;18(10):689-700. doi: 10.1038/s41569-021-00541-4.

[2] Gebreegziabiher G, Belachew T, Mehari K, Tamiru D. Prevalence of dyslipidemia and associated risk factors among adult residents of Mekelle City, Northern Ethiopia. PLoS One 2021;16(2):e0243103. doi: 10.1371/journal.pone.0243103.

[3] World Health Organization. Myanmar: Noncommunicable diseases (NCD) country profiles, 2018. URL: https://www.who.int/nmh/countries/mmr_en.pdf.

[4] Zaw KK, Nwe N, Hlaing SS. Prevalence of cardiovascular morbidities in Myanmar. BMC Res Notes 2017;10(1):99. doi: 10.1186/s13104-017-2422-2.

[5] Htet AS, Kjøllesdal MK, Aung WP, Moe Myint AN, Aye WT, Wai MM, et al. Lipid profiles and determinants of total cholesterol and hypercholesterolemia among 25-74 year-old urban and rural citizens of the Yangon Region, Myanmar: A cross-sectional study. BMJ Open 2017;7(11):e017465. doi: 10.1136/bmjopen-2017-017465.

[6] Pan L, Yang Z, Wu Y, Yin RX, Liao Y, Wang J, et al. The prevalence, awareness, treatment and control of dyslipidemia among adults in China. Atherosclerosis 2016;248:2-9. doi: 10.1016/j.atherosclerosis.2016.02.006.

[7] Pengpid S, Peltzer K. National high prevalence, and low awareness, treatment and control of dyslipidemia among people aged 15-69 years in Mongolia in 2019. Sci Rep 2022;12(1):10478. doi: 10.1038/s41598-022-14729-2.

[8] World Health Organization. STEPwise approach to surveillance (STEPS), 2018. URL: https://www.who.int/ncds/surveillance/steps/en/.

[9] Ministry of Public Health, Myanmar, World Health Organization, World Diabetes Federation. Report on National Survey of Diabetes Mellitus and Risk Factors for Non-communicable Diseases in Myanmar, 2014. URL: https://extranet.who.int/ncdsmicrodata/index.php/catalog/634/download/4544.

[10] World Health Organization. WHO STEPS surveillance manual. URL: https://www.who.int/ncds/surveillance/steps/STEPS_Manual.pdf.

[11] Expert Panel on Detection, Evaluation, and Treatment of High Blood Cholesterol in Adults. Executive summary of the Third Report of the National Cholesterol Education Program (NCEP) Expert Panel on Detection, Evaluation, and Treatment of High Blood Cholesterol in Adults (Adult Treatment Panel III). JAMA 2001;285(19):2486-97. doi: 10.1001/jama.285.19.2486.

[12] Harvard School of Public Health. Abdominal obesity measurement guidelines for different ethnic groups, 2020. URL: https://www.hsph.harvard.edu/obesity-prevention-source/waist-circumference-guidelines-for-different-ethnic-groups/.

[13] Wen CP, David Cheng TY, Tsai SP, Chan HT, Hsu HL, Hsu CC, et al. Are Asians at greater mortality risks for being overweight than Caucasians? Redefining obesity for Asians. Public Health Nutr 2009;12(4):497-506. doi: 10.1017/S1368980008002802.

[14] Chobanian AV, Bakris GL, Black HR, Cushman WC, Green LA, Izzo JL et al. Seventh report of the Joint National Committee of Prevention, Detection, Evaluation, and Treatment of High Blood Pressure. Hypertension 2003;42(6):1206–52. http://dx.doi.org/10.1161/01.HYP.0000107251.49515.c2.

[15] Armstrong T, Bull F. Development of the World Health Organization Global Physical Activity Questionnaire (GPAQ). J Public Health 2006;14:66–70.

[16] Basit A, Sabir S, Riaz M, Fawwad A; NDSP members. NDSP 05: Prevalence and pattern of dyslipidemia in urban and rural areas of Pakistan; A sub analysis from second National Diabetes Survey of Pakistan (NDSP) 2016-2017. J Diabetes Metab Disord 2020;19(2):1215-25. doi: 10.1007/s40200-020-00631-z.

[17] Hong SA, Peltzer K, Lwin KT, Aung S. The prevalence of underweight, overweight and obesity and their related socio-demographic and lifestyle factors among adult women in Myanmar, 2015-16. PLoS One 2018;13(3):e0194454. doi: 10.1371/journal.pone.0194454.

[18] Tähtinen TM, Vanhala MJ, Oikarinen JA, Keinänen-Kiukaanniemi SM. Effect of smoking on the prevalence of insulin resistance-associated cardiovascular risk factors among Finnish men in military service. J Cardiovasc Risk 1998;5(5-6):319-23.

[19] Xi Y, Niu L, Cao N, Bao H, Xu X, Zhu H, et al. Prevalence of dyslipidemia and associated risk factors among adults aged ≥35 years in northern China: A cross-sectional study. BMC Public Health 2020;20(1):1068. doi: 10.1186/s12889-020-09172-9.

[20] Opoku S, Gan Y, Yobo EA, Tenkorang-Twum D, Yue W, Wang Z, et al. Awareness, treatment, control, and determinants of dyslipidemia among adults in China. Sci Rep 2021;11(1):10056. doi: 10.1038/s41598-021-89401-2.

Chapter 11

Prevalence and correlates of sedentary behaviour among adults in Tonga: Trends of national cross-sectional surveys in 2004, 2011, and 2017

Supa Pengpid*, **DrPH**

Department of Health Education and Behavioral Sciences, Faculty of Public Health, Mahidol University, Bangkok, Thailand

Department of Public Health, Sefako Makgatho Health Sciences University, Pretoria, South Africa

Abstract

In this study we aimed to evaluate trends in the prevalence and correlates of low physical activity (PA) and sedentary behaviour (SB) in adults from 2004 to 2017 in Tonga. Cross-sectional data were analysed from 6,961 persons (20-64 years), 907 in 2004, 2,457 in 2011, and 3,597 in 2017 who participated in STEPS surveys in Tonga. Self-reported PA and SB and various health measures were assessed. Overall, 40.1% had low, 24.4% moderate, and 35.5% high PA. The proportion of SB was 26.9% 4 to <8 hours/day and 6.6% ≥8 hours/day. Compared to participants from 2004, participants from 2011 (Adjusted Odds Ratio-AOR: 0.44, 95% confidence interval-CI: 0.37-0.52) had significantly lower odds of low PA. Male sex (AOR: 0.49, 95% CI: 0.43-0.55) decreased the odds and having higher education (≥12 years) (AOR: 1.51, 95% CI: 1.28-1.77) increased the odds of low PA. Inadequate fruit and vegetable intake

* ***Correspondence:*** Professor Supa Pengpid, Department of Health Education and Behavioral Sciences, Faculty of Public Health, Mahidol University, 420/1 Ratchawithi Road, Ratchathewi, Bangkok 10400, Thailand. Email: supaprom@yahoo.com.

In: Non-Communicable Diseases
Editor: Joav Merrick
ISBN: 979-8-89113-514-7

(AOR: 1.68, 95% CI: 1.39-2.04) and having hypertension (AOR: 1.17, 95% CI: 1.04-1.32) were positively associated, and current tobacco smoking (AOR: 0.85, 95% CI: 0.75-0.97) was negatively associated with low PA. Current tobacco smoking (ARRR: 0.73, 95% CI: 0.54-0.98) was negatively associated with high sedentary behaviour (≥8 hours). Higher education (ARRR: 1.26, 95% CI: 1.05-1.53) and high total cholesterol (ARRR: 1.33, 95% CI: 1.07-1.40) were positively associated, and male sex (AOR: 0.79, 95% CI: 0.69-0.91) and overweight (AOR: 0.75, 95% CI: 0.57-0.98) were negatively associated with moderate sedentary behaviour. Two in five adults in Tonga had inadequate PA and one in three had SB. Sociodemographic and health factors were found to be associated with low PA and SB.

Introduction

Physical inactivity has been associated with morbidity and mortality (1, 2). In 2016, among adults, the prevalence of inadequate physical activity (PA) was 27.5% globally, which did not decrease significantly compared to the global prevalence of 2001 (28.5%) (3). We lack data on national trends on PA and sedentary behaviour (SB) in Tonga, an upper middle income country in Oceania (4,5). In Tonga 99.9% of adults are at risk of developing non-communicable diseases, because of high rates of obesity, diabetes, raised cholesterol, smoking and physical inactivity (6).

In Asia, for example, in Iran, the prevalence of inadequate PA increased from 23.1% in 2001 to 55.4% in 2016 (7), in Mongolia the proportion of low PA increased from 10.9% in 2005 to 27.2% in 2013 (9), and in China, SB (>4 hrs/day) increased from 35.4% in 2002 to 43.0% in 2012 (10). In a survey among ageing adults in six countries, including China and India, the prevalence of high SB (≥8 hrs/day) was 8.3% (11).

Sociodemographic risk factors for low PA include increasing age (12), female sex (13), and those with higher education (14). The health factors associated with low PA include obesity (15), hypertension (16), high cholesterol (17), smoking (18), alcohol consumption (19) and poor diet (20). SB may increase with age (21), sex (22, 23), higher socioeconomic status (23), and ethnicity (24). Health factors associated with SB include obesity (≥30 kg/m^2) (11), tobacco use (11, 23), alcohol use (24), and hypertension (24). This study aimed to determine trends in low PA and SB and associated factors among adults from national cross-sectional surveys in 2004, 2011 and 2017 in Tonga.

Our study

Secondary data from cross-sectional STEPS surveys in 2004, 2011, and 2017 in Tonga were analysed (25); the study response rate was 80.0% in 2004, 88.8% in 2011, and 85.7% in 2017 (26-28). "A multi-stage stratified sampling process was carried out to randomly select participants from the target population. An individual per household within the age range of the survey" (15-64 years in 2004, 25-64 in 2011, and 18-69 years in 2017) was included (26-28). The sample in this paper was restricted to participants aged 20-64 years across the three surveys. The Tonga Ministry of Health and the World Health Organization provided approval of the study, and participants gave written informed consent (26-28).

Data collection followed the "WHO three STEPS methodology: Step 1 included the administration of a structured questionnaire (sociodemographics, medical history, medication use, and health risk behaviour), Step 2 consisted of blood pressure and anthropometric measurements, and Step 3 included biochemical tests (blood lipids)" (26-28). A Seca Leicester was used to measure height and the Siltec PS500L was used to measure weight (26-28). Of the three systolic and diastolic blood pressure readings using "OMRON Digital Automatic Blood Pressure Monitor" (26-28); the last two measurements were averaged (26-28). "Total cholesterol was measured in peripheral (capillary) blood at the data collection site using dry chemical methods" (26-28).

Measures

Physical activity was measured using the "Global Physical Activity Questionnaire" (GPAQ) (29), and "calculated from the duration of moderate and vigorous PA (at work, transportation and recreation) in a typical day and week." As per GPAQ guidelines, PA levels were classified as "low, moderate and high" (29).

Sedentary behaviour was sourced from one item of the GPAQ on the "time usually spend sitting or reclining on a typical day?" ("Hours/minutes") (29), and classified as "<4 hours, 4 to <8 hours and ≥8 hours per day" (30).

Other health-risk behaviours included fruit/vegetable consumption (<5 servings/day), current tobacco smoking, and current alcohol use (26-28).

Hypertension defined as “systolic BP ≥140 mm Hg and/or diastolic BP ≥90 mm Hg” (31); raised total cholesterol (TC) (“fasting TC ≥200 mg/dl”).

Body mass index (BMI) was calculated from measured height and weight, and classified as <25 kg/m^2, 25.0-29.9 kg/m^2 (overweight), ≥30.0 kg/m^2 (obesity) (25).

Sociodemographic variables consisted of study year, sex, education, age, and ethnic group (26-28).

Analysis

Unadjusted and adjusted logistic regression was used to assess associations between sociodemographic, health variables, and low PA. Multinomial logistic regression was used to determine the predictors of moderate or high SB (low SB was used as a reference). $p < 0.05$ was considered as significant. “STATA software version 15.0 (Stata Corporation, College Station, TX, USA).” was used for statistical analysis.

Findings

The sample included 6,961 persons (20-64 years), 907 in 2004, 2,457 in 2011, and 3,597 in 2017. Two out of five participants (36.8%) were men and 63.2% women, 43.6% had 12 or more years of education, 99% were Tongan by ethnicity, and 74.4% had obesity. Most (87.7%) had inadequate fruit and vegetable intake, 25.4% were current tobacco smokers, 10.4% were current alcohol users, 34.4% had high total cholesterol, and 30.9% had hypertension. Overall, 40.1% had low, 24.4% moderate, and 35.5% high PA. The proportion of SB was 26.9% 4 to <8 hours/day and 6.6% ≥8 hours/day (see Table 1).

Physical inactivity in the different PA domains

In 2017, 57.9% of the participants reported not vigorous or moderate PA at work, 42.6% did not engage in transport-related activity and 87.6% did not engage in vigorous or moderate PA at leisure-time. This shows that the highest level of PA was reported in the leisure domain. Compared to the study year 2004, the prevalence no PA at work significantly decreased, and no PA in transportation and at leisure-time significantly increased in from 2004 and 2017 (p for trend <0.001). The proportion of no PA at leisure-time, transportation and at work was significantly higher among women than men across study years (see Table 2).

Associations with low PA

In the adjusted logistic regression analysis, compared to participants from 2004, participants from 2011 (Adjusted Odds Ratio-AOR: 0.44, 95% confidence interval-CI: 0.37-0.52) had significantly lower odds of low PA. Male sex (AOR: 0.49, 95% CI: 0.43-0.55) decreased the odds and having higher education (≥12 years) (AOR: 1.51, 95% CI: 1.28-1.77) increased the odds of low PA. Inadequate fruit and vegetable intake (AOR: 1.68, 95% CI: 1.39-2.04), and having hypertension (AOR: 1.17, 95% CI: 1.04-1.32) were positively associated, and current tobacco smoking (AOR: 0.85, 95% CI: 0.75-0.97) was negatively associated with low PA (see Table 3).

Associations with sedentary behaviour

In adjusted multinomial logistic regression, compared to study year 2004, participants in 2017 had higher odds (ARRR: 1.54, 95% CI: 1.27-1.86) of moderate SB (4 to <8 hours per day) and lower odds (ARRR: 0.50, 95% CI: 0.37-0.67) of ≥8 hours SB per day. Current tobacco smoking (ARRR: 0.73, 95% CI: 0.54-0.98) was negatively associated with high SB (≥8 hours). Higher education (ARRR: 1.26, 95% CI: 1.05-1.53) and high total cholesterol (ARRR: 1.33, 95% CI: 1.07-1.40) were positively associated, and male sex (AOR: 0.79, 95% CI: 0.69-0.91) and overweight (AOR: 0.75, 95% CI: 0.57-0.98) were negatively associated with moderate SB (see Table 4).

Discussion

To our knowledge, this is the first investigation to evaluate the trends in prevalence and factors associated with SB among adults in Tonga.

Table 1. Sample, physical activity and sedentary behaviour characteristics, Tonga 2004-2017

Variable	Sample	Physical activity levels			Sedentary behaviour		
		Low	Moderate	High	<4 hours/day	4 to <8 hours/day	≥8 hours/day
	N (%)	%	%	%	%	%	%
All	6961	40.1	24.4	35.5	66.5	26.9	6.6
Study year							
2004	907 (13.0)	43.5	21.9	34.6	67.9	21.0	11.2
2011	2457 (35.3)	25.8	26.2	48.1	71.6	22.5	5.9
2017	3597 (51.7)	49.0	23.9	27.2	62.2	31.9	5.9
Age (years)							
20-34	2073 (29.8)	42.2	23.8	33.9	63.4	30.3	6.3
35-49	3073 (44.1)	39.4	23.5	37.1	67.8	25.8	6.4
50-64	1815 (26.1)	38.9	26.6	34.5	67.8	25.0	7.2
Gender							
Female	4396 (63.2)	46.5	27.7	25.8	64.7	28.6	6.7
Male	2565 (36.8)	29.2	18.8	52.0	69.7	24.0	6.4
Education (in years)							
0-9	1233 (17.8)	33.0	25.7	41.3	70.5	22.2	7.3
10-11	2716 (39.1)	39.5	24.4	36.1	67.6	27.1	5.3
≥12	2990 (43.1)	43.6	24.0	32.5	63.9	28.7	7.5
Ethnic group							
Non-Tongan	62 (1.0)	31.1	26.2	42.6	58.6	37.9	3.4
Tongan	5981 (99.0)	39.7	24.8	35.6	66.4	27.7	5.9
Body mass index							
<25 kg/m^2	474 (7.2)	33.8	21.6	44.6	65.2	29.2	5.7
25-29.9 kg/m^2	1221 (18.5)	32.3	22.6	45.1	70.4	23.7	6.0
≥30 kg/m^2	4920 (74.4)	42.6	25.2	32.2	66.0	27.1	6.8

Variable	**Sample**	**Physical activity levels**			**Sedentary behaviour**		
		Low	**Moderate**	**High**	**<4 hours/day**	**4 to <8 hours/day**	**≥8 hours/day**
	N (%)	%	%	%	%	%	%
Inadequate fruit/ vegetable intake	5826 (87.7)	42.3	24.0	33.8	66.7	27.0	6.3
Current tobacco smoking	1767 (25.4)	31.8	20.8	47.4	69.4	24.9	5.7
Current alcohol use	719 (10.4)	29.8	18.9	51.3	69.5	24.2	6.3
High total cholesterol	2213 (34.4)	39.0	24.1	36.9	65.9	27.5	6.7
Hypertension	2049 (30.9)	44.0	24.5	31.9	65.8	27.4	6.9

Table 2. Physical inactivity by domains of activity

Variable	**2004**	**2011**	**2017**	**p-for trend**
	% (95% CI)	% (95% CI)	% (95% CI)	
All				
No vigorous and no moderate activity at work	62.0 (58.8-65.0)	44.2 (42.2-46.1)	57.9 (56.3-59.5)	0.008
No active transportation	39.3 (36.2-42.5)	32.1 (30.3-34.0)	42.6 (30.3-34.0)	<0.001
No vigorous and no moderate activity at leisure-time	85.0 (82.6-87.1)	78.0 (76.4-79.6)	87.6 (86.6-88.6)	<0.001
Male				
No vigorous and no moderate activity at work	52.2 (47.3-57.1)	30.7 (27.8-33.8)	50.2 (47.5-52.8)	0.004
No active transportation	37.3 (32.7-42.2)	25.8 (23.0-28.7)	39.4 (36.9-42.1)	<0.001
No vigorous and no moderate activity at leisure-time	78.2 (73.4-81.9)	66.6 (63.5-69.6)	80.6 (78.5-82.7)	<0.001
Female				
No vigorous and no moderate activity at work	69.1 (65.1-72.8)	52.4 (49.9-54.9)	62.2 (60.2-64.0)	0.698
No active transportation	40.8 (36.7-44.9)	36.0 (33.6-38.5)	44.3 (42.3-46.2)	<0.001
No vigorous and no moderate activity at leisure-time	90.0 (87.2-92.2)	85.0 (83.1-86.7)	91.5 (0.90-92.5)	<0.001

CI = Confidence interval.

Table 3. Associations between sociodemographic factors, health indicators, and low physical activity estimated by logistic regression in Tonga, 2004-2017

Variable	Crude Odds Ratio (95% CI)	Adjusted Odds Ratio (95% CI)
Study year		
2004	1 (Reference)	1 (Reference)
2011	0.45 (0.39-0.53)***	0.44 (0.37-0.52)***
2017	1.26 (1.09-1.45)**	1.07 (0.91-1.25)
Age (years)		
20-34	1 (Reference)	1 (Reference)
35-49	0.89 (0.79-1.00)*	1.03 (0.90-1.18)
50-64	0.87 (0.76-0.99)*	1.05 (0.90-1.22)
Gender		
Female	1 (Reference)	1 (Reference)
Male	0.48 (0.43-0.53)***	0.49 (0.43-0.55)***
Education (in years)		
0-9	1 (Reference)	1 (Reference)
10-11	1.29 (1.12-1.48)***	1.28 (1.09-1.51)**
≥12	1.50 (1.31-1.72)***	1.51 (1.28-1.77)***
Body mass index		
<25 kg/m^2	1 (Reference)	1 (Reference)
25-29.9 kg/m^2	0.87 (0.70-1.07)	0.86 (0.67-1.09)
≥30 kg/m^2	1.36 (1.13-1.64)***	1.08 (0.86-1.34)
Inadequate fruit/vegetable intake	2.46 (2.07-2.91)***	1.68 (1.39-2.04)***
Current tobacco smoking	0.61 (0.55-0.69)***	0.85 (0.75-0.97)*
Current alcohol use	0.59 (0.50-0.70)	---
High total cholesterol	0.91 (0.82-1.01)	---
Hypertension	1.24 (1.12-1.38)***	1.17 (1.04-1.32)**

CI = Confidence Interval; ***$p < 0.001$; **$p < 0.01$; *$p < 0.05$.

Table 4. Associations between sociodemographic factors, health indicators and sedentary behaviour estimated by multinomial regression in Tonga, 2004-2017

Variable	**Sedentary behaviour in hours a day**	
	4 to <8	**≥8**
	ARRR (95% CI)	**ARRR (95% CI)**
Study year		
2004	1 (Reference)	1 (Reference)
2011	1.01 (0.82-1.24)	0.46 (0.34-0.62)***
2017	1.54 (1.27-1.86)***	0.50 (0.37-0.67)***
Age (years)		
20-34	1 (Reference)	1 (Reference)
35-49	0.86 (0.74-1.00)	1.04 (0.79-1.37)
50-64	0.86 (0.72-1.03)	1.24 (0.90-1.72)
Gender		
Female	1 (Reference)	1 (Reference)
Male	0.79 (0.69-0.91)***	0.86 (0.67-1.10)
Education (in years)		
0-9	1 (Reference)	1 (Reference)
10-11	1.19 (0.99-1.43)	0.77 (0.56-1.06)
≥12	1.26 (1.05-1.53)*	1.24 (0.91-1.69)
Body mass index		
<25 kg/m^2	1 (Reference)	1 (Reference)
25-29.9 kg/m^2	0.75 (0.570.98)*	1.00 (0.59-1.70)
≥30 kg/m^2	0.64-1.03)	1.17 (0.72-1.92)
Inadequate fruit/vegetable intake	1.04 (0.85-1.29)	0.73 (0.53-1.02)
Current tobacco smoking	0.92 (0.79-1.08)	0.73 (0.54-0.98)*
Current alcohol use	1.21 (0.96-1.53)	0.70 (0.43-1.12)
High total cholesterol	1.33 (1.07-1.40)**	0.97 (0.76-1.23)
Hypertension	0.98 (0.85-1.13)	1.11 (0.86-1.42)

CI = Confidence Interval; ***$p < 0.001$; **$p < 0.01$; *$p < 0.05$.

The study found that the proportion of low PA increased (but not significantly) from 2004 (43.5%) to 2017 (49.0%), while in other studies, for example, in Iran low PA increased from 2001 (23.1%) to 2016 (55.4%) (7), and in Mongolia low PA increased from 2005 (10.9%) to 2013 (27.2%) (9). Compared to global estimates (27.5%) the prevalence of low PA in Tonga is high and needs increased intervention efforts (4, 5). Moderate SB increased significantly and high SB decreased significantly from 2004 to 2017 in Tonga, which compares with trend increases of moderate SB in China (10).

Consistent with previous studies (13, 14), the study found a higher prevalence of low PA in women than in men, which means that women should be especially targeted in improving PA. While some studies showed an increase in low PA with age (12), this study did not find a decline in PA with age. In line with previous findings (14), low PA increased with higher education. It is possible that those with higher education status are less likely to participate in PA due to less physical labour. Consistent with previous research (32), this study also found that of the three domains of PA, PA in leisure time was the lowest, highlighting the need to improve infrastructure and accessibility to sports and recreational facilities. Considering that better health can be achieved if PA is spread more evenly in the three PA domains, leisure PA may be strengthened to optimize health (33). Consistent with previous research (23), we found that female sex, and higher education were associated with moderate SB.

In agreement with some research (11, 15-17, 20, 24), we found that health factors, such as hypertension, high cholesterol, inadequate fruit and vegetable consumption, and in unadjusted analysis obesity were associated with low PA and/or moderate SB. Some previous research (11, 18, 23), showed a positive association between smoking and low PA and SB, while we found an inverse association with low PA and SB.

The limitations of the study include the evaluation of some variables by self-report, including PA and SB, and the repeat cross-sectional design. Furthermore, some variables, such as mental health, which could be significantly correlated with PA were not evaluated in all three surveys and therefore were not included in this analysis.

Conclusion

Two in five adults in Tonga had inadequate PA, and one in three had SB. We found that the proportion of low PA did not change significantly between 2004 and 2017. Moderate SB increased significantly, and high SB decreased significantly from 2004 to 2017. Sociodemographic factors (study year, female sex, higher education) and health factors (inadequate fruit and vegetable intake, hypertension, and high cholesterol) were found associated with low PA and/or SB. These identified factors should be considered when designing PA and SB intervention programmes.

Acknowledgments

This paper uses data from the 2004, 2011, and 2017 Tonga STEPS survey, implemented by the Tonga Ministry of Health with the support of the World Health Organization.

References

[1] World Health Organization. Reducing risks, promoting healthy life. World Health Report 2002. Geneva: WHO, 2002.

[2] Vancampfort D, Koyanagi A, Ward PB, Rosenbaum S, Schuch FB, Mugisha J, et al. Chronic physical conditions, multimorbidity and physical activity across 46 low- and middle-income countries. Int J Behav Nutr Phys Act 2017;14(1):6. doi: 10.1186/s12966-017-0463-5.

[3] Guthold R, Stevens GA, Riley LM, Bull FC. Worldwide trends in insufficient physical activity from 2001 to 2016: a pooled analysis of 358 population-based surveys with 1·9 million participants. Lancet Glob Health 2018;6(10):e1077-86. doi: 10.1016/S2214-109X(18)30357-7.

[4] Turk T, Latu N, Cocker-Palu E, Liavaa V, Vivili P, Gloede S, et al. Using rapid assessment and response to operationalise physical activity strategic health communication campaigns in Tonga. Health Promot J Austr 2013;24(1):13-9. doi: 10.1071/HE12903.

[5] Keane L, Sherry E, Schulenkorf N, Negin J, Ding D, Bauman A, et al. Personal, social, and environmental mediators associated with increased recreational physical activity in women and girls in the Kingdom of Tonga. J Phys Act Health 2020;17(11):1100-8. doi: 10.1123/jpah.2019-0630.

[6] Tonga Health. National strategy to prevent and control non-communicable diseases 2015- 2020. Nuku'alofa, Tonga: Tonga Health Promotion Foundation. URL: https://www.dfat.gov.au/sites/default/files/tonga-national-non-communicable-disease-strategy-2015-20.pdf.

[7] Kamalian A, Khosravi Shadmani F, Yoosefi M, Mohajer B, Mohebi F, Naderimagham S, et al. A national and sub-national meta regression of the trend of

insufficient physical activity among Iranian adults between 2001 and 2016. Sci Rep 2021;11(1):21441. doi: 10.1038/s41598-021-00252-3.

[8] Aryal KK, Mehata S, Neupane S, Vaidya A, Dhimal M, Dhakal P, et al. The burden and determinants of non-communicable diseases risk factors in Nepal: Findings from a Nationwide STEPS survey. PLoS One 2015;10(8):e0134834. doi: 10.1371/journal.pone.0134834.

[9] Dashzeveg D, Nakamura K, Seino K, Al-Sobaihi S, Palam E. Changes in the configuration and patterns of physical activity among Mongolian adults, 2005-2013. J Rural Med 2018;13(2):151-9. doi: 10.2185/jrm.2977.

[10] Ding C, Feng G, Yuan F, Gong W, Yao Y, Ma Y, et al. Temporal trends and recent correlates in sedentary behaviors among Chinese adults from 2002 to 2010-2012. Int J Environ Res Public Health 2019;17(1):158. doi: 10.3390/ijerph17010158.

[11] Koyanagi A, Stubbs B, Vancampfort D. Correlates of sedentary behavior in the general population: A cross-sectional study using nationally representative data from six low- and middle-income countries. PLoS One 2018;13(8):e0202222. doi: 10.1371/journal.pone.0202222.

[12] Moniruzzaman M, Mostafa Zaman M, Islalm MS, Ahasan HA, Kabir H, Yasmin R. Physical activity levels in Bangladeshi adults: Results from STEPS survey 2010. Public Health 2016;137:131-8. doi: 10.1016/j.puhe.2016.02.028.

[13] Bauman AE, Reis RS, Sallis JF, Wells JC, Loos RJ, Martin BW; Lancet Physical Activity Series Working Group. Correlates of physical activity: Why are some people physically active and others not? Lancet 2012;380(9838):258-71. doi: 10.1016/S0140-6736(12)60735-1.

[14] Devamani CS, Oommen AM, Mini G K, Abraham VJ, George K. Levels of physical inactivity in rural and urban Tamil Nadu, India: A cross-sectional study. J Clin Prev Cardiol 2019;8:13-7

[15] World Health Organization. Overweight and obesity, 2021. URL: https://www.who.int/news-room/fact-sheets/detail/obesity-and-overweight.

[16] de Ramirez SS, Enquobahrie DA, Nyadzi G, Mjungu D, Magombo F, Ramirez M, Sachs SE, Willett W. Prevalence and correlates of hypertension: a cross-sectional study among rural populations in sub-Saharan Africa. J Hum Hypertens 2010;24(12):786-95. doi: 10.1038/jhh.2010.14.

[17] Milton K, Macniven R, Bauman A. Review of the epidemiological evidence for physical activity and health from low- and middle-income countries. Glob Public Health 2014;9(4):369-81. doi: 10.1080/17441692.2014.894548.

[18] Bennie JA, Pedisic Z, van Uffelen JG, Gale J, Banting LK, Vergeer I, et al. The descriptive epidemiology of total physical activity, muscle-strengthening exercises and sedentary behaviour among Australian adults--results from the National Nutrition and Physical Activity Survey. BMC Public Health 2016;16:73. doi: 10.1186/s12889-016-2736-3.

[19] Jakkaew N, Pinyopornpanish K, Jiraporncharoen W, Wisetborisut A, Jiraniramai S, Hashmi A, et al. Risk of harm from alcohol use and heavy alcohol consumption: Its association with other NCD risk factors in Thailand. Sci Rep 2019;9(1):16343. doi: 10.1038/s41598-019-52754-w.

[20] Koyanagi A, Stubbs B, Smith L, Gardner B, Vancampfort D. Correlates of physical activity among community-dwelling adults aged 50 or over in six low- and middle-income countries. PLoS One 2017;12(10):e0186992. doi: 10.1371/journal.pone.0186992.

[21] Müller AM, Chen B, Wang NX, Whitton C, Direito A, Petrunoff N, et al. Correlates of sedentary behaviour in Asian adults: A systematic review. Obes Rev 2020;21(4):e12976. doi: 10.1111/obr.12976.

[22] Tcymbal A, Andreasyan D, Whiting S, Mikkelsen B, Rakovac I, Breda J. Prevalence of Physical Inactivity and Sedentary Behavior Among Adults in Armenia. Front Public Health 2020;8:157. doi: 10.3389/fpubh.2020.00157.

[23] Dendup T, Zhao Y, Edi Putra IGN. Correlates of sedentary behavior among Bhutanese adults: Findings from the 2014 Bhutan STEPS Survey Data. Korean J Fam Med 2021;42(4):288-96. doi: 10.4082/kjfm.20.0059.

[24] Peltzer K, Phaswana-Mafuya, Pengpid S. Prevalence and correlates of sedentary behaviour among a national sample of 15-98 years old individuals in South Africa. AJPHES 2018;24(3):286-98.

[25] Motuma A, Gobena T, Roba KT, Berhane Y, Worku A. Sedentary behavior and associated factors among working adults in Eastern Ethiopia. Front Public Health 2021;9:693176. doi: 10.3389/fpubh.2021.693176.

[26] World Health Organization. STEPwise approach to surveillance (STEPS), 2018. URL: https://www.who.int/ncds/surveillance/steps/en/.

[27] World Health Organization. Kingdom of Tonga NCD Risk Factors STEPS Report 2004. Suva: World Health Organization, 2012. URL: https://extranet.who.int/ncdsmicrodata/index.php/catalog/721/related-materials.

[28] World Health Organization. Kingdom of Tonga NCD Risk Factors STEPS Report 2012. Suva: World Health Organization, 2014. URL: https://extranet.who.int/ncdsmicrodata/index.php/catalog/717/related-materials.

[29] World Health Organization (WHO). STEPS Tonga 2017, Factsheet. URL: ttps://extranet.who.int/ncdsmicrodata/index.php/catalog/713/related-materials.

[30] Armstrong T, Bull F. Development of the World Health Organization Global Physical Activity Questionnaire (GPAQ). J Public Health 2006;14:66–70.

[31] Ekelund U, Steene-Johannessen J, Brown WJ, Fagerland MW, Owen N, Powell KE, et al. Does physical activity attenuate, or even eliminate, the detrimental association of sitting time with mortality? A harmonised meta-analysis of data from more than 1 million men and women. Lancet 2016;388(10051):1302-10. doi: 10.1016/S0140-6736(16)30370-1.

[32] Chobanian AV, Bakris GL, Black HR, Cushman WC, Green LA, Izzo JL et al. Seventh report of the Joint National Committee of Prevention, Detection, Evaluation, and Treatment of High Blood Pressure. Hypertension 2003;42(6):1206–52. http://dx.doi.org/10.1161/01.HYP.0000107251.49515.c2.

[33] Strain T, Wijndaele K, Garcia L, Cowan M, Guthold R, Brage S, et al. Levels of domain-specific physical activity at work, in the household, for travel and for leisure among 327 789 adults from 104 countries. Br J Sports Med 2020;54(24):1488-97. doi: 10.1136/bjsports-2020-102601.

[34] Pedišić Ž, Dumuid D, Olds T. Integrating sleep, sedentary behaviour, and physical activity research in the emerging field of time-use epidemiology: Definitions, concepts, statistical methods, theoretical framework, and future directions. Kinesiology 2017;49:252–69.

Chapter 12

The association between soft drink consumption and health risk behaviors among school-going adolescents in Bolivia

Zuchi Lkhamsuren[1], MSc
Karl Peltzer[1,2,*], PhD
Passakorn Suanrueang[3], PhD
and Lyen Krenz Yap[1], RPm, MSc

[1]Department of Psychology, College of Medical and Health Science, Asia University, Taiwan
[2]Department of Psychology, University of the Free State, Bloemfontein, South Africa
[3]Department of Healthcare Administration Specialty in Psychology, College of Medical and Health Science, Asia University, Taiwan

Abstract

In this chapter we aim to study the relationship between soft drink consumption (SDC) and health risk behaviors among =11 years to =18 years old Bolivian students. The secondary analysis of the cross-sectional 2018 Bolivia Global School-Based Student Health Survey was used. The sample included 7,931 adolescents (50.3% males, and 49.7% females), mean age 15.5 years (SD = 1.6). The study found that no or <once/day SDC in the past 7 days was 66.3%, once a day 15.2%, two or three times a day 12.1%, and four or more times per day 6.4% (33.7% at least once per day). Students who had one to three times soft drinks per day were

* *Correspondence:* Karl Peltzer, Department of Psychology, College of Medical and Health Science, Asia University, Wufeng, Taichung 41354, Taiwan; Email: kfpeltzer@gmail.com.

In: Non-Communicable Diseases
Editor: Joav Merrick
ISBN: 979-8-89113-514-7

more likely to have been injured (OR: 1.27, 95% CI: 1.09, 1.48; OR: 1.30, 95% CI: 1.08, 1.56), Students who drank two or more soft drinks a day were more likely to engage in a physical fight in the last 12 months. (OR: 1.41, 95% CI: 1.19, 1.69; OR: 1.35, 95% CI: 1.07, 1.70), current alcohol use (OR: 1.41, 95% CI: 1.16, 1.71; OR: 1.59, 95% CI: 1.21, 2.08), students who drank four or more soft drinks a day were more likely to attempt suicide (OR: 1.30, 95% CI: 1.02, 1.64), sat for 3 or more hours per day during leisure time (OR: 1.51, 95% CI: 1.25, 1.82), been ever drunk (OR: 1.61, 95% CI: 1.23, 2.11), and cyberbullied (OR: 1.43, 95% CI: 1.03, 1.99). There was no relationship between SDC and physical inactivity, current cannabis use, physically attacked, amphetamine use, and bullied in or outside the school. Soft drink consumption was associated with eight of 13 health risk behaviors.

Introduction

Sugar intake is associated with individual health risk behaviors (physical fights, bullying, smoking, drinking, and drunkenness) in 26 industrialized countries (1). Carbonated soft drinks are the main source of added sugar in the selection of foods (2). The use of tobacco, fast food, and alcohol by Ghanaian high school students was associated with increased consumption of soft drinks (3). In the study of the association between sugar-containing soft drink consumption (SDC) and conduct problems in school-going adolescents in Oslo, Norway, the highest odds ratio was observed between both genders who drank more than four glasses of soft drinks per day (4). A study on adolescents in the United States found an association between SDC and other factors relating to psychological distress, such as feeling sad or hopeless and experiencing suicidal ideation (5). Moreover, being attacked, physical injury, being involved in a physical fight, academic truancy and lifetime drunkenness (6), inadequate sleep, sedentary behavior, and cigarette smoking (7), not always wearing a seatbelt, being bullied, being injured within school property, and relationship-related violence (8), alcohol (6), marijuana and amphetamines (9) were significantly associated with higher SDC. The meta-analysis of GSBS Survey concluded that carbonated SDC was high in Latin America countries and, of 18 countries, Bolivia was the 9th highest SDC country (10). In the study of Bolivian 13-17 years old school adolescents, 34.3% in the plains and 30.1% in the valley regions' students were consuming =1 glass of soft drinks per day (11). Despite the multitude of studies that explore the significant relationship between SDC and health risk behaviors, along with a significant rise of SDC being seen among Bolivian adolescents, there are a lack of cross-sectional studies which investigate the association between SDC and health risk behaviors among Bolivian adolescents. This study aims to study the relationship between SDC and health risk behaviors among =11 years to =17 years old Bolivian students.

Our study

This study used a secondary analysis of the cross-sectional 2018 Bolivia Global School-Based Student Health Survey (N = 7,931) and a "two-stage cluster sample design was used to produce data representative of all students in 2nd Secondary - 6th Secondary in Bolivia" (12). Firstly, educational institutions were primarily chosen with probability proportional to enrollment size (12). Second, classes were randomly selected and each student was able to participate in the survey (12). Response rates were as follows: 94% for the school, 84% for the students, and 79% overall (12). The study was approved by the Ministry of Health, Bolivia, and a national ethics committee, and the "necessary approvals and permission, including informed consent, were obtained from the participating schools, the parents, and the students before the survey was administered" (12).

Measures

The measure used in this survey was the Global School Health Survey 2018, which included demographic information of the respondents and a variety of topics related to SDC (12). The details of all the questions used in the survey are described in Table 1.

Exposure variable

SDC was assessed with the question, "During the past seven days, how many times did you drink a can, bottle, or glass of a carbonated soft drink, such as Pepsi, Coca-Cola, Fanta, Papaya Salvieti or Kinoto? (Do not include diet soft drinks.)" Response options included: "1) I did not drink carbonated soft drinks during the past seven days, 2) 1 to 3 times during the past seven days, 3) 4 to

6 times during the past seven days, 4) 1 time per day, 5) Twice per day, 6) Three times per day, 7) Four or more times per day" Responses were coded 1-3 = <once/day, 4 = once/day, 5-6 = 2-3 times per day, 7 = 4 or more times per day.

Outcome variables

Outcome variables included suicide attempt, physical inactivity, sitting 3 or more hours, ever being drunk, current cannabis use, current alcohol use, amphetamine use, physically attacked, physical fighting, injury, bullied at school, bullied outside school, cyberbullied.

Analysis

Descriptive statistics were employed to show tabulations. Logistic regression was used to measure odds ratios (with 95% confidence interval = CI) for each outcome of risk behavior separately. The final model was adjusted for socio-economic status (hunger), age, sex, school attendance, and parental and peer support. Both the confidence interval and p-value were statistically adjusted for the multi-stage sampling and weighting of the data. Data missing were omitted from the analysis. All statistical procedures were calculated using the STATA software version 15.0 (Stata Corporation, College Station, TX, USA).

Our findings

In the cross-sectional GSHS, the study's sample consisted of 7,931 Bolivian adolescents (50.3% males, and 49.7% females), with a mean age of 15.5 years (SD = 1.6). In terms of SCD, the study found that more than half of the respondents (66.3%) had none or less than once per day in the past seven days. 33.7% of the sample drank soft drinks at least once a day, 15.2% once a day, 12.1% two or three times a day and 6.4% four or more times a day (see Table 2).

Table 1. Variable description

Variables	Question	Response option
Age	"How old are you?"	"11 years old or younger to 18 years old or older"
Sex	"What is your sex?"	Male, Female
Hunger	"During the past 30 days, how often did you go hungry because there was not enough food in your home?"	"1 = never to 5 = always (coded 1–3 = 0 and 4–5 = 1)"
Exposure variable		
Soft drinks	"During the past 7 days, how many times did you drink a can, bottle, or glass of a carbonated soft drink, such as Pepsi, Coca-Cola, Fanta, Papaya Salvieti or Kinoto?"	"1 = not in the past days to 7 = 4 or more times per day (coded 1-2 = 1, 3 = 2, 4-5 = 3 and 6-7 = 4)"
Health risk behaviors		
Suicide attempt	"During the past 12 months, how many times did you actually attempt suicide?"	"1 = 0 times to 5 = 6 or more times (coded 1 = 0 and 2–5 = 1)"
Physically inactive	"During the past 7 days, on how many days were you physically active for a total of at least 60 minutes per day?"	"1 = 0 days to 8 = 7 days (coded 1 – 6 = 0 and 7 = 1)"
Sitting ≥3 hours	"How much time do you spend during a typical or usual day sitting and watching television, playing computer games, talking with friends, or doing other sitting activities such as playing with the mobile phone or videogames?"	"1 = less than 1 hour to 6 = more than 8 hours (coded 1 - 3 = 0 and 4 – 6 = 1)"
Ever drunk	"During your life, how many times did you drink so much alcohol that you were really drunk?"	"1=0 times to 4= 10 or more times (coded 1=0 and 2-4=1)"
Cannabis currently	"During the past 30 days, how many times have you used marijuana (also called marijuana, yerba, or mota)?"	"1 = 0 times to 5 = 20 or more times (coded 1 = 0 and 2 – 5 = 1)"
Physically attacked	"During the past 12 months, how many times were you physically attacked?"	"1 = 0 times to 8 = 12 or more times (coded 1 = 0 and 2 - 8 = 1)"
Physical fighting	"During the past 12 months, how many times were you in a physical fight?"	"1 = 0 times to 8 = 12 or more times (coded 1 = 0 and 2 – 8 = 1)"
Injured	"During the past 12 months, how many times were you seriously injured?"	"1 = 0 times to 8 = 12 or more times (coded 1 = 0 and 2 – 8 = 1)"

Table 1. (Continued)

Variables	Question	Response option
Current alcohol use	"During the past 30 days, on how many days did you have at least one drink containing alcohol?"	"1 = 0 days to 7 = all 30 days (coded 1 = 0 and 2 - 7 = 1)"
Amphetamine	"During your life, how many times have you used amphetamines or methamphetamines (also called pastillas or pepas)?"	"1 = 0 days to 5 = 20 or more times (coded 1 = 0 and 2 – 5 = 1)"
Bullied in school	"During the past 12 months, have you ever been bullied on school property?"	"1 = yes to 2 = no (coded 2 = 0 and 1 = 1)"
Bullied outside school	"During the past 12 months, have you ever been bullied when you were not on school property?"	"1 = yes to 2 = no (coded 2 = 0 and 1 = 1)"
Cyberbullied	"During the past 12 months, have you ever been cyberbullied?"	"1 = yes to 2 = no (coded 2 = 0 and 1 = 1)"
Confounding factors		
School attendance	"During the past 30 days, on how many days did you miss classes or school without permission?"	"1 = 0 days to 5 = 10 or more days (coded 1 = 0 and 2 – 5 = 1)"
Peer support	"During the past 30 days, how often were most of the students in your school kind and helpful?"	"1 = never to 5 = always (coded 1 – 3 = 0 and 4 – 5 = 1)"
Parental support	"During the past 30 days, how often did your parents or guardians understand your problems and worries?"	"1 = never to 5 = always (coded 0 – 1 = low, 2 = medium, 3 – 5 = high)"

Table 2. Sample characteristics and soft drink consumption (SDC) frequency among adolescents in Bolivia, 2018

Variable	Sample	SDC in the past 7 days			
		<once/day	Once/day	2-3 times/day	≥4 times/day
	n (%)	**n (%)**	**n (%)**	**n (%)**	**n (%)**
Sociodemographic					
All	7931 (100)	5226 (66.3)	1186 (15.2)	936 (12.1)	503 (6.4)
Gender					
Male	4014 (50.7)	2647 (66.3)	602 (15.0)	460 (11.7)	274 (6.9)
Female	3763 (49.3)	2503 (66.6)	561 (15.3)	452 (12.3)	216 (5.8)
Age (years)					
11-≤14	2366 (30.5)	1495 (64.2)	380 (16.1)	302 (12.9)	162 (6.8)
15	1593 (20.4)	1057 (66.3)	247 (16.0)	190 (12.0)	87 (5.7)
16	1591 (19.9)	1078 (68.6)	222 (14.0)	183 (11.6)	91 (5.8)
17+	2286 (29.3)	1556 (67.5)	322 (14.3)	250 (11.6)	147 (6.6)
Hunger	317 (4.1)	186 (59.2)	49 (16.1)	43 (13.7)	34 (11.0)
Health risk behaviors					
Suicide attempt	1610 (21.8)	1007 (62.6)	257 (16.0)	217 (13.3)	129 (8.1)
Physically inactive	6553 (88.7)	4332 (65.8)	1008 (15.5)	804 (12.4)	409 (6.3)
Sitting 3 or more hours	2333 (31.6)	1543 (65.8)	298 (12.8)	294 (12.9)	198 (8.6)
Ever drunk	1783 (24.1)	1135 (63.5)	252 (14.1)	238 (13.6)	158 (8.9)
Cannabis currently	561 (7.8)	349 (62.1)	89 (16.8)	71 (12.4)	52 (8.7)
Physically attacked	2187 (28.6)	1400 (64.0)	325 (15.0)	305 (13.7)	157 (7.3)
Physical fighting	2337 (30.6)	1454 (62.5)	355 (15.2)	340 (14.5)	188 (7.8)
Injured	3708 (52.1)	2360 (63.3)	589 (16.2)	504 (13.6)	255 (6.9)
Current alcohol use	1970 (26.4)	1234 (62.3)	279 (14.4)	284 (14.5)	173 (8.7)
Amphetamine use	304 (4.5)	181 (60.5)	49 (16.4)	49 (15.3)	25 (7.7)
Bullied in school	1804 (24.7)	1169 (64.5)	291 (16.0)	213 (12.3)	131 (7.2)
Bullied outside school	1624 (21.7)	1032 (63.2)	274 (16.9)	204 (13.1)	114 (6.9)
Cyberbullied	1601 (21.4)	1012 (62.9)	261 (16.5)	193 (12.4)	135 (8.2)

Table 2. (Continued)

Variable	**Sample**	**SDC in the past 7 days**			
		<once/day	**Once/day**	**2-3 times/day**	**≥4 times/day**
	n (%)	**n (%)**	**n (%)**	**n (%)**	**n (%)**
Confounding factors					
School attendance	4444 (59.2)	3023 (67.9)	676 (15.2)	486 (11.0)	259 (6.0)
Peer support	2598 (34.4)	1752 (67.4)	390 (15.1)	302 (11.6)	154 (5.9)
Parental support					
Low (0-1)	3621 (51.6)	2400 (65.9)	548 (15.3)	428 (12.0)	245 (6.8)
Medium (2)	1584 (22.0)	1048 (65.8)	227 (14.4)	210 (13.4)	99 (6.3)
High (3-4)	1883 (26.3)	1263 (67.1)	309 (16.4)	205 (10.8)	106 (5.7)

Table 3. Associations between soft drink consumption (SDC) frequency and health risk behaviors

SDC in the past 7 days	COR	AOR1
	Suicide attempt	*Suicide attempt*
<once day	1 (Reference)	1 (Reference)
Once/day	1.14 (0.92, 1.40)	1.06 (0.83, 1.35)
2-3 times/day	1.19 (0.98, 1.44)	1.11 (0.92, 1.35)
≥4 times/day	1.44 (1.15, 1.79)**	1.30 (1.02, 1.64)*
	Physically inactive	*Physically inactive*
<once day	1 (Reference)	1 (Reference)
Once/day	1.10 (0.86, 1.41)	1.11 (0.87, 1.42)
2-3 times/day	1.20 (0.95, 1.50)	1.18 (0.94, 1.49)
≥4 times/day	0.80 (0.56, 1.13)	0.79 (0.57, 1.12)
	Sitting more than 3 hours	*Sitting more than 3 hours*
<once day	1 (Reference)	1 (Reference)
Once/day	.77 (0.63, 0.93)**	0.78 (.64, 0.95)
2-3 times/day	1.10 (0.93, 1.29)	1.07 (0.91, 1.26)
≥4 times/day	1.56 (1.31, 1.87)***	1.51 (1.25, 1.82)***
	Ever drunk	*Ever drunk*
<once day	1 (Reference)	1 (Reference)
Once/day	.93 (0.79, 1.10)	0.92 (0.75, 1.12)
2-3 times/day	1.22 (0.97, 1.53)	1.22 (0.97, 1.53)
≥4 times/day	1.65 (1.31, 2.09)***	1.61 (1.23, 2.11)***
	Cannabis currently	*Cannabis currently*
<once day	1 (Reference)	1 (Reference)
Once/day	1.19 (0.89, 1.60)	1.21 (0.91, 1.61)
2-3 times/day	1.11 (0.84, 1.46)	0.94 (0.67, 1.31)
≥4 times/day	1.51 (1.09, 2.11)*	1.35 (0.89, 2.05)
	Physically attacked	*Physically attacked*
<once day	1 (Reference)	1 (Reference)
Once/day	1.02 (0.86, 1.18)	0.97 (0.82, 1.15)
2-3 times/day	1.24 (1.06, 1.44)**	1.12 (0.94, 1.32)
≥4 times/day	1.23 (1.01, 1.51)*	1.11 (0.91, 1.37)
	Physical fighting	*Physical fighting*
<once day	1 (Reference)	1 (Reference)
Once/day	1.08 (0.90, 1.29)	1.07 (.89, 1.30)
2-3 times/day	1.42 (1.21, 1.67)***	1.41 (1.19, 1.69)***
≥4 times/day	1.45 (1.17, 1.78)***	1.35 (1.07, 1.70)**
	Injured	*Injured*
<once day	1 (Reference)	1 (Reference)
Once/day	1.27 (1.10, 1.46)***	1.27 (1.09, 1.48)**
2-3 times/day	1.40 (1.21, 1.62)***	1.30 (1.08, 1.56)**
≥4 times/day	1.33 (1.07, 1.64)**	1.24 (0.98, 1.56)
	Current alcohol use	*Current alcohol use*
<once day	1 (Reference)	1 (Reference)
Once/day	0.99 (0.87, 1.13)	.95 (0.81, 1.11)
2-3 times/day	1.40 (1.15, 1.70)***	1.41 (1.16, 1.71)***
≥4 times/day	1.67 (1.30, 2.15)***	1.59 (1.21, 2.08)***

Table 3. (Continued)

SDC in the past 7 days	COR	AOR1
	Suicide attempt	Suicide attempt
	Amphetamine	*Amphetamine*
<once day	1 (Reference)	1 (Reference)
Once/day	1.18 (0.86, 1.61)	1.11 (0.82, 1.51)
2-3 times/day	1.40 (1.03, 1.91)*	1.01 (0.64, 1.60)
≥4 times/day	1.34 (0.84, 2.16)	0.83 (0.48, 1.45)
	Bullied in school	*Bullied in school*
<once day	1 (Reference)	1 (Reference)
Once/day	1.11 (0.94, 1.31)	1.04 (0.88, 1.23)
2-3 times/day	1.08 (0.93, 1.25)	1.00 (0.87, 1.16)
≥4 times/day	1.25 (1.01, 1.54)*	1.12 (0.89, 1.42)
	Bullied outside school	*Bullied outside school*
<once day	1 (Reference)	1 (Reference)
Once/day	1.21 (1.03, 1.43)*	1.15 (0.97, 1.37)
2-3 times/day	1.19 (1.02, 1.38)*	1.09 (0.90, 1.32)
≥4 times/day	1.16 (0.88, 1.51)	1.00 (0.74, 1.35)
	Cyberbullied	*Cyberbullied*
<once day	1 (Reference)	1 (Reference)
Once/day	1.19 (1.02, 1.38)*	1.16 (0.97, 1.38)
2-3 times/day	1.12 (0.92, 1.36)	1.05 (0.82, 1.34)
≥4 times/day	1.46 (1.09, 1.95)**	1.43 (1.03, 1.99)*

[1]Adjusted for age, sex, hungry (proxy of low economic status), school attendance, peer support, parental support; ***P < 0.001, **P < 0.01, *P < 0.05. COR: Crude Odds Ratio; AOR: Adjusted Odds Ratio.

Associations with soft-drink consumption

In the final adjusted logistic regression analysis, compared to students who had considerably less soft-drink consumption ("never or less than once per day") for the past seven days, students with high soft-drink intake ("one to three times per day") were more likely to have been physically injured (OR: 1.27, 95% CI: 1.09, 1.48; OR: 1.30, 95% CI: 1.08, 1.56), students who had an even higher frequency of soft-drink consumption ("two or more times per day") were more likely to have engaged in a physical fight for the past 12 months (OR: 1.41, 95% CI: 1.19, 1.69; OR: 1.35, 95% CI: 1.07, 1.70), and consumed alcohol in the past month (OR: 1.41, 95% CI: 1.16, 1.71; OR: 1.59, 95% CI: 1.21, 2.08). Students with the highest frequency of soft drink consumption ("four or more times per day") were more likely to have attempted suicide (OR: 1.30, 95% CI: 1.02, 1.64), sat for 3 or more hours per day during leisure time (OR: 1.51, 95% CI: 1.25, 1.82), have been drunk (OR:

1.61, 95% CI: 1.23, 2.11), and have been cyberbullied (OR: 1.43, 95% CI: 1.03, 1.99). There was no significant association between SDC and physical inactivity, current cannabis use, physically attacked, amphetamine use, and bullied in or outside school (see Table 3).

Discussion

This study provides new information on the relationship between SDC and health risk behaviors among adolescents in Bolivian schools. One third of the study's sample (prevalence of 33.7%) drank at least one soft drink a day. This study found a consistent association between higher frequency of SDC and health risk behaviors (injured, physically attacked, participation in physical fighting, current alcohol use, suicide attempt, sitting more than 3 hours, ever drunk, and cyberbullied).

The prevalence of SDC (=1 per day) (33.7%) among adolescents in Bolivia, which is lower than the global prevalence of 42.8% (10), lower than in Latin America (65.1%) (13), similar to Ghana (34. 9%) (3) and lower than in Bolivia in 2012 (63%) (13). The findings of this study regarding the connection between SDC and health risk behaviors are consistent with previous studies in school going adolescents in Europe (physical fight, and alcohol use) (1), USA (in terms of sedentary behavior, being bullied, injured, and physically hurt (7, 8), Southeast Asia (in terms of attacked, injury, physical fight, being bullied, alcohol use, lifetime drunkenness, and suicide attempts) (6), and Seychelles (in terms of being physically attacked, being involved in a physical fight, physical injury, being bullied, current alcohol use, lifetime drunkenness, and suicide attempt) (14).

Using problem behavior theory (15), we could conceptualize that SDC is interrelated with other problem behaviors, such as peer violence and drug use. The consumption of soft drinks is accompanied by a variety of health-risk behaviors, indicating that the school's public health program needs to pay more attention on this topic regarding improving students' understanding of SDC and its negative effect on their health behaviors. (16) found that adolescents' sugar sweetened beverage intake, including soft drinks, is associated with their parents' consumption of it. Therefore, future studies could explore the parents soft drink consumption and interventions focused on parents may be helpful in reducing SDC among adolescents in Bolivia. In addition, explorations of other potential influencing factors, such as smartphone usage (17), of higher SDC among adolescents in Bolivia are necessary.

Study limitation

The study was cross-sectional, which refutes the causal conclusion. The measured variables were self-reported and may be under-reported. Several research indicators were evaluated in single item, and more comprehensive measures should be used for further research.

Conclusion

One in three adolescents in Bolivia consumes soft drinks at least once a day. This study extends previous studies from high-income countries and Asia that a consistent association between higher frequency of SDC and health risk behaviors (injured physically attacked, participation in physical fights, current alcohol use, suicide attempt, sitting more than 3 hours, ever drunk and cyberbullied) was found in South America (Bolivia). Relevant suggestions regarding school policies are explored.

Acknowledgments

This paper uses data from the Global School-Based Student Health Survey (GSHS). GSHS is supported by the World Health Organization and the US Centers for Disease Control and Prevention.

References

[1] Bruckauf Z, Walsh SD. Adolescents' multiple and individual risk behaviors: Examining the link with excessive sugar consumption across 26 industrialized countries. Soc Sci Med 2018;216:133-41. doi: 10.10 16/j.socscimed.2018.08.029.

[2] Harrington S. The role of sugar-sweetened beverage consumption in adolescent obesity: A review of the literature. J Sch Nurs 2008;24(1):3-12. doi: 10.1177/10598405080240010201.

[3] Atorkey P, Akwei M, Asare-Doku W. Consumption of carbonated soft drinks among Ghanaian adolescents: associations with socio-demographic factors, health risk factors and psychological distress. Nutr Health 2021;27(3):329-36. doi: 10.1177/0260106021996933.

[4] Lien L, Lien N, Heyerdahl S, Thoresen M, Bjertness E. Consumption of soft drinks and hyperactivity, mental distress, and conduct problems among adolescents in

Oslo, Norway. Am J Public Health 2006;96(10):1815-20. doi: 10.2105/AJPH.2004.059477.

[5] Solnick SJ, Hemenway D. Soft drinks, aggression and suicidal behaviour in US high school students. Int J Inj Contr Saf Promot 2014;21(3):266-73. doi: 10.1080/17457300.2013.815631.

[6] Pengpid S, Peltzer K. High carbonated soft drink intake is associated with health risk behavior and poor mental health among school-going adolescents in six Southeast Asian Countries. Int J Environ Res Public Health 2019;17(1):132. doi: 10.3390/ijerph17010132.

[7] Park S, Sherry B, Foti K, Blanck HM. Self-reported academic grades and other correlates of sugar-sweetened soda intake among US adolescents. J Acad Nutr Diet 2012;112(1):125-31. doi: 10.1016/j.jada.2011.08.045.

[8] Park S, Blanck HM, Sherry B, Foti K. Problem behavior, victimization, and soda intake in high school students. Am J Health Behav 2013;37(3):414-21. doi: 10.5993/AJHB.37.3.14.

[9] Terry-McElrath YM, O'Malley PM, Johnston LD. Energy drinks, soft drinks, and substance use among United States secondary school students. J Addict Med 2014;8(1):6-13. doi: 10.1097/01.ADM.0000435322.07020.53.

[10] Beal T, Morris SS, Tumilowicz A. Global patterns of adolescent fruit, vegetable, carbonated soft drink, and fast-food consumption: A meta-analysis of global school-based student health surveys. Food Nutr Bull 2019;40(4):444-59. doi: 10.1177/0379572119848287.

[11] Villalta N, Arauco N, Mamani M, Illanes DE, Singh P, Moura LD, et al. Dietary patterns among 13-17-years old school adolescents: A national comparison of the three geographical regions in Bolivia. medRxiv 2021. https://doi.org/10.1101/2021.07.22.21259344.

[12] Bolivia (Plurinational State of)—Global School-Based Student Health Survey, 2018. URL: https://extranet.who.int/ncdsmicrodata/index.php/catalog/881.

[13] Yang L, Bovet P, Liu Y, Zhao M, Ma C, Liang Y, Xi B. Consumption of carbonated soft drinks among young adolescents aged 12 to 15 years in 53 low- and middle-income countries. Am J Public Health 2017;107(7):1095-1100. doi: 10.2105/AJPH.2017.303762.

[14] Pengpid S, Peltzer K. High carbonated soft drink consumption is associated with externalizing and internalizing behaviour among in-school adolescents in the Seychelles. Int J Child Adolesc Health 2019;12(2):213-21.

[15] Jessor R. Problem behavior and psychosocial development: A longitudinal study of youth. New York: Academic Press, 1977.

[16] Lundeen EA, Park S, Onufrak S, Cunningham S, Blanck HM. Adolescent sugar-sweetened beverage intake is associated with parent intake, not knowledge of health risks. Am J Health Promot 2018;32(8):1661-70. doi: 10.1177/0890117118763008.

[17] Ryu S, Jang H, Oh H. Smartphone usage patterns and dietary risk factors in adolescents. J Nutr 2022;152(9):2109-16.

Chapter 13

Non-communicable disease risk factors and non-work participation among older adults in India

Karl Peltzer[*], **PhD**

Department of Psychology, University of the Free State, Bloemfontein, South Africa
Department of Psychology, College of Medical and Health Science, Asia University, Taichung, Taiwan

Abstract

Non-communicable diseases risk factors may influence work participation among older adults. The aim of this study was to assess the determinants of non-work participation among older adults in India. The national sample consisted of 31,447 individuals (≥60 years) in India. Work participation was assessed with the question, "Are you currently working." In total, 69.2% were not and 30.8% were working. Older age, female sex, not married, high socioeconomic status, not reserved caste, urban residence, not food insecurity, hypertension, heart disease or stroke, chronic lung disease, diabetes, polypharmacy, physical inactivity, functional limitations, impaired vision, impaired hearing, poor/fair self-rated health status, and not currently using tobacco were associated with non-work participation. Almost one in three older adults in India are working. Factors associated with a non-working status included sociodemographic and health factors, which may in part be addressed in public health interventions.

---

[*] ***Correspondence:*** Karl Peltzer, Department of Psychology, College of Medical and Health Science, Asia University, Wufeng, Taichung 41354, Taiwan.
Email: kfpeltzer@gmail.com.

In: Non-Communicable Diseases
Editor: Joav Merrick
ISBN: 979-8-89113-514-7

Introduction

India is a rapidly ageing country (1, 2), with having 34% of older adults (≥60 years) participating in the labour force (3-5). The "older population in India is affected by non-communicable diseases, including chronic lung conditions, cardiovascular diseases, stroke, cancer, multiple disabilities, vision and hearing problems, mental health problems, and cognitive impairment" (6).

According to the World Health Organization, ten key determinants of work participation among older adults include "labour market, legislation and its implementation, financial, social position, domestic, human resources, work, health, work ability, and motivation" (7, 8). Work participation in other low resourced countries, such as Brazil, found that among older adults (≥60 years), the proportion of work participation was 16.7% (9), and in the USA (≥65 years), 21% (10).

Sociodemographic factors associated with non-participation in work among older adults include increased age (9, 11), female sex (9-12), lower education (9), lower socioeconomic status (13), higher education (12), higher socioeconomic status in India (3), no health insurance (14) and urban residence (12). Physical chronic conditions associated with non-participation in work among older adults include number of physical chronic conditions, multimorbidity (11), diabetes (15), arthritis (15) and polypharmacy (11). Functional and sensory limitations associated with non-participation in work among older adults include lower physical functioning (10, 16, 17), physical inactivity (13), low hand grip strength (11) and poor visual perception (11). Mental health conditions associated with non-participation in work among older adults include poor self-rated health (9, 12, 14, 18, 19), poorer cognitive functioning (16, 20), poorer mental health (PHQ-4 scores) (10), depression (15), lower depression (18, 20), not geriatric depression (21), lower life satisfaction (20) and not smoking (13).

There is a lack of national population-based data on the social and health determinants of work participation among older adults in India. Therefore, the aim of this study was to assess determinants non-work participation in older community-dwelling adults in India. It would be important to understand the determinants of non-work participation among older adults in India to improve public health care planning.

Our study

This secondary data analysis used data from the cross-sectional "Longitudinal Ageing Study in India (LASI) Wave 1, 2017-2018"; "the overall household response rate is 96%, and the overall individual response rate is 87%." (22). In a household survey, "interview, physical measurement and biomarker data were collected from individuals aged 45 and above and their spouses, regardless of age" (22), but the sample was restricted to persons 60 years and older. The study was approved by the "Indian Council of Medical Research (ICMR) Ethics Committee in January 2017 and written or oral informed consent was obtained from the participants" (23).

Measures

Work status was sourced from two questions, 1) "Are you currently working?" (Yes/No) and 2) "Have you ever worked for at least 3 months during your lifetime? Work includes agricultural work, wage work, self-employed activities, and unpaid family business work. Work also includes all kinds of labor, excluding doing your own housework, whether you earn wages or not." (22).

Covariates

Sociodemographic information included subjective socioeconomic status, health insurance, age, education, sex, caste and residence status (22).

Food insecurity was defined from any positive response to four questions: 1) "In the last 12 months, did you ever reduce the size of your meals or skip meals because there was not enough food at your household? (Yes/No) 2) In the last 12 months, were you hungry but didn't eat because there was not enough food at your household? (Yes/No) 3) In the past 12 months, did you ever not eat for a whole day because there was not enough food at your household? 4) Do you think that you have lost weight in the last 12 months because there was not enough food in your household?" (22).

Physical chronic conditions were sourced from the questions, "Has any health professional ever told you that you have...?": 1) "chronic lung diseases such as asthma, chronic obstructive pulmonary disease/chronic bronchitis or other chronic lung problems; 2) chronic heart diseases such as coronary heart disease (heart attack or myocardial infarction), congestive heart failure, or other chronic heart problems; 4) diabetes or high blood sugar; 5) bone or joint disorder (arthritis or rheumatism, Osteoporosis or other bone/joint diseases); and 6) stroke." (Yes/No) (22). *Hypertension or raised blood pressure (BP)* was defined as "systolic BP ≥140 mm Hg and/or diastolic BP ≥90 mm Hg (based on the last two averaged of three BP readings) or where the participant is currently on antihypertensive medication." (23). "Body mass index=BMI was calculated according to Asian criteria: underweight (<18.5 kg/m^2), normal weight (18.5-22.9 kg/m^2), overweight (23.0-24.9 kg/m^2), class I obesity (25.0-29.9 kg/m^2), and class II obesity (≥30.0 kg/m^2)" (24).

Medication use was assessed for the treatment of ten conditions (Yes/No), as follows: "1) In order to control your blood pressure or hypertension, are you currently taking any medication? 2) During the last two years, did you take medications and treatments for symptoms (pain, nausea, rashes) of cancer? 3) Are you currently taking any medication for your heart disease? 4) Are you currently taking any medication or receiving other treatments for your arthritis, rheumatism, or osteoporosis? 5) Are you currently taking tranquilizers, antidepressants, or other types of medication for neurological or psychiatric problem(s)? 6) Do you take analgesics (oral/ injectable) to get relief from the pain? 7) Are you currently taking any medications because of your stroke or its complications? 8) Do you regularly take medications to help lower your cholesterol? 9) In the past 1 month, have you taken any medications or used other treatments to help you sleep? 10) In order to treat or control your diabetes or high blood sugar, are you currently taking medications that you swallow?" (22). The ten uses of medications were summed and trichotomized into 1=0, 2=1-3 and 3=4-8 medications.

Major injury was assessed with the question, "In the past two years, have you sustained any major injuries?" (Yes/No) (22).

Physical activity (PA) was assessed with questions on the frequency and time of participation in moderate or vigorous physical activities (22), and classified into 4 levels of PA (no, low, moderate and high) (25, 26).

Functional disability was sourced from "Activities of Daily Living (ADL) (6 items) and Instrumental Activities of Daily Living (IADL) (7 items)" (27, 28).

Impaired vision was defined as "self-reported poor or very poor far and near eyesight despite use of corrective lenses," and *hearing impairment* as "having diagnosed with any hearing or ear-related problem or condition" (22).

Impaired cognition was classified based on a series of cognitive tests (22, 29).

Self-rated health status was sourced from the item, "In general, would you say your health is excellent, very good, good, fair, or poor?" (22).

Depressive symptoms (≥4 scores) were defined based on the Centre for Epidemiological Studies Depression Scale (CES-D-10) (30).

Insomnia symptoms were assessed with the Jenkins Sleep Scale (JSS-4) (32-34).

Neurological or psychiatric disorder (health care provider diagnosed any "neurological, or psychiatric problems such as depression, Alzheimer's/Dementia, unipolar/bipolar disorders, convulsions, Parkinson's, etc." (Yes, No) (22).

Current tobacco use included, 1) "Do you currently smoke any tobacco products (cigarettes, bidis, cigars, hookah, cheroot, etc.)? and/or 2) Do you use smokeless tobacco (such as chewing tobacco, gutka, pan masala, etc.)?" (22).

Analysis

Descriptive statistics were applied to describe the sample. Chi-square tests were used to test differences in proportions. Logistic regressions were used to estimate the predictors of non-work participation. Variables significant in univariable analysis were subsequently included in the multivariable model. $P < 0.05$ was accepted as significant. Statistical analyses were conducted using "STATA software version 15.0 (Stata Corporation, College Station, TX, USA)," taking the complex study design into account.

Findings

The sample consisted of 31,447 older adults (≥60 years), 39.1% had low subjective socioeconomic status, 18.2% had health insurance, 10.5% had food insecurity and 74.2% belonged to reserved castes. Half of the participants (49.8%) had hypertension, 14.3% diabetes, 19.7% bone or joint disease, 8.5% chronic lung disease, 7.6% heart disease or stroke, 26.9% underweight, 35.3% overweight/obesity, 1.9% polypharmacy use, and 15.1% major injury. Two in five older adults (41.4%) had functional limitations, 47.7% were physically inactive, 13.7% had impaired vision, and 9.6% had impaired hearing. Almost half of the participants (48.6%) rated their health status as fair or poor, 9.3% had impaired cognition, 30.2% had depressive symptoms, 14.8% had insomnia symptoms, 2.8% had a neurological or psychiatric disorder, and 33.7% were currently using tobacco. In all, 69.2% were not and 30.8% were working. Among those who work, 58.0% worked in the agricultural sector, 18.3% were self-employed, 6.4% assisted in non-agricultural work, and 27.2% received a salary (see Table 1).

Table 1. Sample and working participation characteristics among older adults (≥60 years) in India, 2017-2018 (N = 31,447)

Variable	Sample	Working	Not working	Odds Ratio (95% CI)	p-value
	%	%	%		
Sociodemographic factors					
All		30.8	69.2		
Age in years					
60-69	58.5	40.8	59.2	1 (Reference)	
70 plus	41.5	16.7	83.3	3.45 (3.12, 3.81)	<0.001
Gender					
Male	47.5	43.8	56.2	1 (Reference)	
Female	52.5	19.0	81.0	3.33 (3.03, 3.65)	<0.001
Education					
1 year or more	43.5	31.9	68.1	1 (Reference)	
No schooling	56.5	29.9	70.1	1.09 (0.98, 1.22)	0.104
Marital status					
Not married	38.4	19.2	80.8	1 (Reference)	
Married	61.6	37.9	62.1	0.39 (0.35, 0.44)	<0.001
Socioeconomic status					
Low	39.1	35.0	65.0	1 (Reference)	
Medium	36.7	32.4	67.6	1.13 (1.01, 1.25)	0.033
High	24.2	24.4	75.6	1.67 (1.49, 1.88)	<0.001
Caste					
Unreserved	25.8	24.1	75.9	1 (Reference)	
Reserved	74.2	33.2	66.8	0.64 (0.58, 0.71)	<0.001
Residential status					
Rural	70.5	30.8	64.6	1 (Reference)	
Urban	29.5	19.6	80.4	2.25 (1.95, 2.60)	<0.001
Food insecurity					
No	89.5	30.3	69.7	1 (Reference)	
Yes	10.5	35.4	64.6	0.79 (0.68, 0.92)	0.002
Has health insurance	18.2	35.9	64.1	0.76 (0.67, 0.85)	<0.001
Physical chronic conditions					
Hypertension	49.8	25.7	74.3	1.64 (1.54, 1.75)	<0.001
Heart disease or stroke	7.6	16.1	83.9	2.83 (2.42, 3.32)	<0.001
Chronic lung disease	8.5	20.8	79.2	1.74 (1.50, 1.99)	<0.001
Bone or joint disorder	19.7	22.9	77.1	1.74 (1.63, 1.87)	<0.001
Diabetes	14.3	19.1	80.9	2.00 (1.74, 2.31)	<0.001

Variable	Sample	Working	Not working	Odds Ratio (95% CI)	p-value
	%	%	%		
General body weight					
Normal	37.9	35.6	64.4	1 (Reference)	
Underweight	26.9	34.2	65.8	1.06 (0.96, 1.18)	0.219
Overweight/obesity	35.3	26.1	73.9	1.56 (1.39, 1.76)	<0.001
Medication use					
None	52.8	38.6	61.4	1 (Reference)	
1-3	45.3	23.0	77.0	1.99 (1.88, 2.11)	<0.001
4-8	1.9	8.2	91.8	7.43 (4.87, 11.34)	<0.001
Major injury	15.1	27.7	72.3	1.17 (1.06, 1.28)	0.002
Physical functional, and sensory limitations					
Physical activity					
None	33.3	13.7	86.3	1 (Reference)	
Low	14.4	29.6	70.4	0.38 (0.33, 0.44)	<0.001
Moderate	8.4	27.6	72.4	0.42 (0.35, 0.50)	<0.001
High	43.9	44.8	55.2	0.20 (0.17, 0.22)	<0.001
Functional limitations	41.4	19.1	80.9	2.74 (1.45, 3.06)	<0.001
Impaired vision	13.7	18.5	81.5	2.16 (1.82, 2.57)	<0.001
Impaired hearing	9.6	20.2	79.8	1.86 (1.57, 2.20)	<0.001
Mental health					
Impaired cognition	9.3	20.4	79.6	2.10 (1.85, 2.39)	<0.001
Poor or fair self-rated health	48.6	26.2	73.8	1.69 (1.56, 1.83)	<0.001
Depressive symptoms	30.2	28.1	71.9	1.25 (1.12, 1.40)	<0.001
Insomnia symptoms	14.8	24.6	75.4	1.44 (1.27, 1.63)	<0.001
Neurological or psychiatric disorder	2.8	20.4	79.6	2.00 (1.69, 2.37)	<0.001
Current tobacco use	33.7	43.4	56.6	0.43 (0.41, 0.46)	<0.001

Associations non-work participation

In adjusted logistic regression analysis, sociodemographic factors (older age, female gender, not married, high socioeconomic status, not reserved caste, urban residence, and not food insecurity) were associated with non-work participation. In terms of health factors, hypertension, heart disease or stroke, chronic lung disease, diabetes, polypharmacy, physical inactivity, functional limitations, impaired vision, impaired hearing, poor/fair self-rated health status, and not currently using tobacco were associated with non-work participation (see Table 2). In addition, in unadjusted analysis, having no health insurance, overweight/obesity, major injury, impaired cognition, depressive symptoms, insomnia symptoms, and having a neurological or psychiatric disorder were associated with non-work participation (see Table 2).

Table 2. Associations with non-work participation

Variable	Adjusted Odds Ratio (95% CI)	p-value
Sociodemographic factors		
Age in years		
60-69	1 (Reference)	
70 plus	2.63 (2.32, 2.98)	<0.001
Gender		
Male	1 (Reference)	
Female	3.97 (3.53, 4.46)	<0.001
Marital status		
Not married	1 (Reference)	
Married	0.83 (0.72, 0.94)	0.005
Socioeconomic status		
Low	1 (Reference)	
Medium	1.04 (0.92, 1.17)	0.533
High	1.57 (1.36, 1.82)	<0.001
Caste		
Unreserved	1 (Reference)	
Reserved	0.62 (0.53, 0.74)	<0.001
Residential status		
Rural	1 (Reference)	
Urban	1.87 (1.63, 2.15)	<0.001
Food insecurity		
No	1 (Reference)	
Yes	0.68 (0.56, 0.82)	<0.001
Has health insurance	0.96 (0.85, 109)	0.549
Health factors		
Physical chronic conditions		
Hypertension	1.16 (1.04, 1.29)	0.009
Heart disease or stroke	1.42 (1.11, 1.82)	0.005
Chronic lung disease	1.77 (1.46, 2.14)	<0.001
Bone or joint disorder	1.05 (0.91, 1.21)	0.499
Diabetes	1.32 (1.08, 1.61)	0.006
General body weight		
Normal	1 (Reference)	
Under	1.09 (0.97, 1.23)	0.160
Over/obesity	1.07 (0.95, 1.22)	0.275
Medication use		
None	1 (Reference)	
1-3	1.27 (1.12, 1.45)	<0.001
4-8	1.86 (1.09, 2.98)	0.021
Major injury	1.13 (0.97, 1.31)	0.131

Variable	Adjusted Odds Ratio (95% CI)	p-value
Functional and sensory limitations		
Physical activity		
None	1 (Reference)	
Low	0.46 (0.39, 0.54)	<0.001
Moderate	0.46 (0.38, 0.56)	<0.001
High	0.21 (0.18, 0.24)	<0.001
Functional limitations	1.49 (1.31, 1.68)	<0.001
Impaired vision	1.52 (1.25, 1.84)	<0.001
Impaired hearing	1.21 (1.00, 1.47)	0.046
Mental health		
Impaired cognition	1.20 (0.99, 1.47)	0.069
Poor or fair self-rated health	1.30 (1.17, 1.45)	<0.001
Depressive symptoms	1.03 (0.90, 1.17)	0.687
Insomnia symptoms	1.15 (0.98, 1.34)	0.078
Neurological or psychiatric problem	0.93 (0.67, 1.29)	0.660
Current tobacco use	0.75 (0.67, 0.84)	<0.001

Discussion

To our knowledge, this study is the first to determine factors associated with non-work participation among older adults in India. This study found a work participation of 30.8%, which is lower than estimates of older adults (≥60 years) in India in 2012/2013 (34%) (5), but higher than in a study in four Brazilian cities (16.7%, ≥60 years) (9), and in USA (21%, ≥65 years) (10).

Consistent with previous research (3, 9-12), increasing age, female sex, higher socioeconomic status, and residing in urban areas was associated with non-work participation. Some previous research (9, 12, 14) showed that lower or higher education and not having health insurance were associated non-work participation, while we did not find any significant association between educational level and work participation, and in univariable analysis, receipt of health insurance was protective against non-work participation. Furthermore, as expected, food insecurity and belonging to reserved castes increased the odds of work participation. Regarding sex differences, women had a higher probability of non-work participation than men, which can be attributed in part to "excluding doing your own housework" as work participation. Additionally, women may have a higher burden of chronic physical diseases that can hinder their participation in work (11, 35). Policies that support the participation of women in the workforce are indicated. Older adults with lower socioeconomic status, belonging to reserved castes, food insecurity, and living in rural areas were more likely to participate in work, reflecting their deprived social and economic background that calls for public policy intervention for the social security of older adults in India (3).

In terms of physical chronic conditions, this study showed that hypertension, heart disease or stroke, chronic lung disease, diabetes, and polypharmacy were associated with non-work participation. These findings are in line with previous studies (11, 15) showing an association between the number of physical chronic conditions, multimorbidity, diabetes, arthritis and polypharmacy. Older adults who took more medications reflecting the treatment of multiple conditions may have poorer health, preventing them from participating in work (11).

Consistent with previous studies (10, 11, 13, 16, 17), this study found that physical inactivity, functional limitations, impaired vision, and impaired hearing increased the odds of non-work participation. It is possible that through participation in work physical activity increases and functional limitations decrease (11, 13). Sensory deficits, such as impaired vision and hearing, may limit mobility and impact negatively on activities at the workplace (11).

In line with a number of previous studies (9, 10, 12, 14), this study showed an association between poor or fair self-rated health status and non-work participation. While several previous studies (10, 15, 16, 20), found an association between poor mental health, poor cognition, and non-work participation, we only found in univariate analysis an association between impaired cognition, depressive symptoms, insomnia symptoms, neurological or psychiatric disorder and non-work participation. Moreover, in agreement with a previous study (13), this survey found that not currently using tobacco was associated with non-work participation.

The limitations of the study include the cross-sectional design and the evaluation of some variables by self-report.

Conclusion

Almost one in three older adults in India are working. Factors associated with non-work participation included sociodemographic factors (older age, female gender, not married, high socioeconomic status, not reserved caste, urban residence, and not food insecurity) and health factors (having hypertension, heart disease or stroke, chronic lung disease, diabetes, polypharmacy, physical inactivity, functional limitations, impaired vision, impaired hearing, poor or fair self-rated health status, and not currently using tobacco). Public health interventions may address musculoskeletal and cardiorespiratory capacity, food security and physical activity health promotion.

Acknowledgments

The Longitudinal Aging Study in India Project is funded by the Ministry of Health and Family Welfare, Government of India, the National Institute on Aging (R01 AG042778, R01 AG030153), and United Nations Population Fund, India.

References

[1] United Nations Population Fund (UNPFA). India 2018. URL: https://www.unfpa.org/sites/default/files/IN_UNFPA_Results_07_27.pdf .

[2] United Nations Population Fund (UNPFA). Caring for our elders: Early responses - India Ageing Report 2017. New Delhi: UNFPA, 2017. URL: https://india.unfpa.org/sites/default/files/pub-pdf/India%20Ageing%20Report%20-%202017%20%28Final%20Version%29.pdf .

[3] Reddy AB. Labour force participation of elderly in India: Patterns and determinants. Int J Soc Econ 2016;43(5):502-16.

[4] Age Discrimination Info. Retirement age in India: demographic timebomb means changes will be needed to deal with ageing population, 2019. URL: http://www.agediscrimination.info/news/2019/7/15/retirement-age-in-india.

[5] NSSO. Key indicators of employment and unemployment in India, NSS 68th Round (July 2011–June 2012). New Delhi: National Sample Survey Office, Ministry of Statistics and Programme Implementation, Government of India, 2013. URL: http://mospi.nic.in/sites/default/files/publication_reports/KI-68th-E%26U-PDF.pdf.

[6] Malik C, Khanna S, Jain Y, Jain R. Geriatric population in India: Demography, vulnerabilities, and healthcare challenges. J Fam Med Prim Care 2021;10(1):72-6. doi: 10.4103/jfmpc.jfmpc_1794_20.

[7] World Health Organization. Decade of healthy ageing: Baseline report. Geneva: World Health Organization, 2020.

[8] Federal Ministry of Labour and Social Affairs. Understanding employment participation of older workers: defining research needs for evidence-based policy. Berlin: Federal Ministry of Labour and Social Affairs, 2015. URL: https://www.jp-demographic.eu/wp-content/uploads/2015/07/JPIUEP_Brochure1.pdf.

[9] Castro CMS, Costa MFL, Cesar CC, Neves JAB, Sampaio RF. Influence of education and health conditions on paid work of elderly Brazilians. Cien Saude Colet 2019;24(11):4153-62. doi: 10.1590/1413-812320182411.05762018.

[10] Marfeo EE, Ward C. Older adult productive activity participation using the National Health and Aging Trends Study. Gerontol Geriatr Med 2020;6:2333721420910657. doi: 10.1177/2333721420910657.

[11] Dantas RG, Perracini MR, Guerra RO, Ferriolli E, Dias RC, Padula RS. What are the sociodemographic and health determinants for older adults continue to participate in work? Arch Gerontol Geriatr 2017;71:136-41. doi: 10.1016/j.archger.2017.04.005.

[12] Bakshi S, Prasanta P. *Who works at older ages? the correlates of economic activity and temporal changes in their effects: evidences from India. I*n: Yadava AK. Ageing: some emerging issues - Profiles, trends and policy perspectives. New Delhi: Manak Publications, 2011:253-78.

[13] Amorim JS, Salla S, Trelha CS. Factors associated with work ability in the elderly: systematic review. Rev Bras Epidemiol 2014;17(4):830-41. doi: 10.1590/1809-4503201400040003.

[14] Ling DC, Chi I. Determinants of work among older adults in urban China. Australas J Ageing 2008;27(3):126-33. doi: 10.1111/j.1741-6612.2008.00307.x.

[15] Yen L, McRae I, Jeon YH, Essue B, Herath P. The impact of chronic illness on workforce participation and the need for assistance with household tasks and personal care by older Australians. Health Soc Care Community 2011;19(5):485-94. doi: 10.1111/j.1365-2524.2011.00994.x.

[16] Li J, Yuan B, Lan J. The influence of late retirement on health outcomes among older adults in the policy context of delayed retirement initiative: an empirical attempt of clarifying identification bias. Arch Public Health 2021;79(1):59. doi: 10.1186/s13690-021-00582-8.

[17] Santos KA, Koszuoski R, Dias-da-Costa JS, Pattussi MP. Factors associated with functional incapacity among the elderly in Guatambu, Santa Catarina State, Brazil. Cad Saude Publica 2007;23(11):2781-8. doi: 10.1590/s0102-311x2007001100025.

[18] Li Y, Xu L, Chi I, Guo P. Participation in productive activities and health outcomes among older adults in urban China. Gerontologist 2014;54(5):784-96. doi: 10.1093/geront/gnt106.

[19] Schwingel A, Niti MM, Tang C, Ng TP. Continued work employment and volunteerism and mental well-being of older adults: Singapore longitudinal ageing studies. Age Ageing 2009;38(5):531-7. doi: 10.1093/ageing/afp089.

[20] Gladius Jennifer H, Bagavandas M. Determinants of depression status of elderly in Kancheepuram District: A community based neighborhood study. Indian J Public Health Res Dev 2020;11(7):1209-14.

[21] International Institute for Population Sciences (IIPS), NPHCE, MoHFW, Harvard TH Chan School of Public Health (HSPH) and the University of Southern California (USC). Longitudinal Ageing Study in India (LASI) Wave 1, 2017-18, India Report. Mumbai: nternational Institute for Population Sciences, 2020.

[22] Chobanian AV, Bakris GL, Black HR, Cushman WC, Green LA, Izzo Jr JL, et al. The seventh report of the joint national committee on prevention, detection, evaluation, and treatment of high blood pressure: the JNC 7 report. JAMA 2003;289(19):2560–71

[23] Wen CP, David Cheng TY, Tsai SP, Chan HT, Hsu HL, et al. Are Asians at greater mortality risks for being overweight than Caucasians? Redefining obesity for Asians. Public Health Nutr 2009;12(4):497-506. doi: 10.1017/S1368980008002802.

[24] World Health Organization (WHO). WHO guidelines on physical activity and sedentary behaviour. Geneva: World Health Organization, 2020.

[25] Huffman MD, Capewell S, Ning H, Shay CM, Ford ES, Lloyd-Jones DM. Cardiovascular health behavior and health factor changes (1988-2008) and projections to 2020: Results from the National Health and Nutrition Examination Surveys. Circulation 2012;125(21):2595-602. doi: 10.1161/CIRCULATIONAHA.111.070722.

[26] Katz S, Ford AB, Moskowitz RW, Jackson BA, Jaffe MW. Studies of illness in the aged. the index of adl: a standardized measure of biological and psychosocial function. JAMA 1963;185:914-9. doi: 10.1001/jama.1963.03060120024016.

[27] Lawton MP, Brody EM. Assessment of older people: Self-maintaining and instrumental activities of daily living. Gerontologist 1969;9(3):179-86.

[28] Lee J, Smith JP. Regional disparities in adult height, educational attainment and gender difference in late-life cognition: Findings from the Longitudinal Aging Study in India (LASI). J Econ Ageing 2014;4:26-34. doi: 10.1016/j.jeoa.2014.02.002.

[29] Andresen EM, Malmgren JA, Carter WB, Patrick DL. Screening for depression in well older adults: evaluation of a short form of the CES-D (Center for Epidemiologic Studies Depression Scale). Am J Prev Med 1994;10(2):77-84.

[30] Kumar S, Nakulan A, Thoppil SP, Parassery RP, Kunnukattil SS. Screening for depression among community-dwelling elders: Usefulness of the Center for Epidemiologic Studies Depression Scale. Indian J Psychol Med 2016;38(5):483-5. doi: 10.4103/0253-7176.191380.

[31] Jenkins CD, Stanton BA, Niemcryk SJ, Rose RM. A scale for the estimation of sleep problems in clinical research. J Clin Epidemiol 1988;41(4):313-21. doi: 10.1016/0895-4356(88)90138-2.

[32] Cho E, Chen TY. The bidirectional relationships between effort-reward imbalance and sleep problems among older workers. Sleep Health 2020;6(3):299-305. doi: 10.1016/j.sleh.2020.01.008.

[33] Fabbri M, Beracci A, Martoni M, Meneo D, Tonetti L, Natale V. Measuring subjective sleep quality: A review. Int J Environ Res Public Health 2021;18(3):1082. doi: 10.3390/ijerph18031082.

[34] Oztürk A, Simşek TT, Yümin ET, Sertel M, Yümin M. The relationship between physical, functional capacity and quality of life (QoL) among elderly people with a chronic disease. Arch Gerontol Geriatr 2011;53(3):278-83. doi: 10.1016/j.archger.2010.12.011.

Chapter 14

National cross-sectional data on undiagnosed type 2 diabetes among adults in Ecuador

Supa Pengpid*, DrPH
Department of Health Education and Behavioral Sciences, Faculty of Public Health, Mahidol University, Bangkok, Thailand
Department of Public Health, Sefako Makgatho Health Sciences University, Pretoria, South Africa

Abstract

This chapter aim to assess the prevalence and associated factors of undiagnosed type 2 diabetes (T2D) among adults in Ecuador. Cross-sectional data (N = 4,040, 18-69 years) who participated in the Ecuador STEPS survey in 2018, who had complete fasting blood glucose measurement. The prevalence of undiagnosed T2D was 3.7% (3.6% of total T2D), diagnosed T2D 6.7%, and total T2D 10.4%. In the adjusted multinomial logistic regression analysis, older age (50-69 years) (ARRR: 7.93, 95% CI: 3.49-18.04), obesity (ARRR: 1.90, 95% CI: 1.14-3.14), and elevated total cholesterol (ARRR: 2.05, 95% CI: 1.40-3.00) were positively associated with undiagnosed T2D versus no T2D. Older age (50-69 years) (ARRR: 5.70, 95% CI: 2.61-12.45), health care visit (ARRR: 3.12, 95% CI: 2.12-4.57), obesity (ARRR: 1.56, 95% CI: 1.02-2.40), hypertension (ARRR: 1.52, 95% CI: 1.11-2.08), and elevated total cholesterol (ARRR: 1.60, 95% CI: 1.18-2.18) were positively associated with diagnosed T2D versus no T2D. In the logistic regression analysis, only the health care visit (AOR: 0.27, 95% CI: 0.16-0.47) was negatively associated with undiagnosed T2D versus diagnosed T2D. A significant

* *Correspondence:* Professor Supa Pengpid, Department of Health Education and Behavioral Sciences, Faculty of Public Health, Mahidol University, 420/1 Ratchawithi Road, Ratchathewi, Bangkok 10400, Thailand. Email: supaprom@yahoo.com.

In: Non-Communicable Diseases
Editor: Joav Merrick
ISBN: 979-8-89113-514-7

proportion of adults in Ecuador had undiagnosed T2D, and several associated factors were identified which can help in guiding interventions.

Introduction

According to the World Health Organization (1), an "estimated 1.5 million deaths are directly caused by diabetes in 2019; diabetes can be treated, and its consequences avoided or delayed with diet, physical activity, medication and regular screening and treatment for complications." Untreated and undiagnosed type 2 diabetes (T2D) can have serious consequences, including microvascular and macrovascular complications (2, 3) and an increased risk of mortality (4, 5), highlighting the crucial importance of early diagnosis. In 2021, "almost one in two adults (20–79 years old) with T2D were unaware of their T2D status (44.7%)" (6). In an earlier review of studies in 29 low- and middle-income countries (LMICs), the prevalence of undiagnosed T2D was 4.9% (7). For example, in Suriname, 39.6% of people with T2D had not been previously diagnosed (8), in northern Sudan among people with T2D 29.0% were newly diagnosed (9), in a health clinic on Santa Cruz Island, Ecuador, the prevalence of undiagnosed diabetes was 11% (n = 16) (10), and among adults in China, the prevalence of undiagnosed T2D was 6.9% (63.3% of total T2D) (11). There is lack of national data on undiagnosed T2D in Ecuador (12), which led to the study.

Factors associated with undiagnosed T2D can be grouped into predisposing, enabling and need factors (13, 14), including younger age (15-17), older age (13, 18-20), lower among age ≥ 70 years vs. 35-39 years (21), male sex (16-18), living alone (17, 22), marital or cohabitation status (22), ethnic minority (23), ethnicity (24), and family history of diabetes (25, 26). Enabling/disabling factors may include lower economic status (15, 21), food insecurity (27), lower education (16, 28), rural residence (13, 15), geographical regions (13, 16, 17, 29), know symptoms of diabetes (25), no recent health care visit (17), health insurance status (13, 30), and health risk behaviours (high sedentary behaviour (12), heavy alcohol use (31), high level of physical activity (21), and fitness compared to peers (19). The need factors may include hypertension status [not hypertension (15, 16), hypertension (18, 19, 31, 32)], obesity (18-20, 25, 26, 31, 33), low HDL-C (33, 34), high triglycerides (33, 34), dyslipidaemia (26), cardiovascular disease status [not heart disease (16), cardiovascular disease (19)], and poor perceived health

(13). The study aimed to estimate the prevalence and associated factors of undiagnosed T2D among people (15-69 years) in Ecuador.

Our study

Secondary data from the 2018 Ecuador STEPS (35) with complete measurements of fasting blood glucose were analysed. Following the STEPS survey procedures, "Socio-demographic and behavioural information was collected in Step 1. Physical measurements such as height, weight, and blood pressure were collected in Step 2. Biochemical measurements were collected to assess blood glucose and cholesterol levels in Step 3" (35).

"A multi-stage stratified sampling process was carried out to randomly select participants from the target population (18 -69 years)" (36). The study was approved by the Ecuador Ministry of Health Ethical Committee, and participants gave written informed consent.

Measures

Undiagnosed T2D was defined as "fasting plasma glucose level ≥126 mg/dL among people who responded 'no' the question 'Have you ever been told by a doctor or other health worker that you have raised blood sugar or diabetes?'" (35).

Predisposing factors: age, sex, ethnicity, and marital status.

Enabling factors: health care visit in the past 12 months, smoking (current and past), past month heavy alcohol use (≥6 units in a single drinking occasion), and physical activity levels (37).

Need factors: body mass index (BMI), hypertension, heart attack or stroke, and high total cholesterol. BMI was classified as "underweight (<18.5 kg/m^2), normal weight (18.5-24.9 kg/m^2), overweight (25.0-29.9 kg/m^2), and obesity (≥30.0 kg/m^2)" (35). Hypertension was defined as "systolic BP ≥140 mmHg and/or diastolic BP ≥90 mmHg and/or previously or current treatment with antihypertensive drugs" (38). Self-reported heart attack or stroke: "Have you ever had a heart attack or chest pain from heart disease (angina) or a stroke (cerebrovascular accident or incident)? (Yes, No)" (36). High total cholesterol was classified (39) as: "being on antilipidemic medication or having elevated total cholesterol (TC): ≥5.17 mmol/l (200 mg/dl)."

Analysis

All statistical analyses were conducted with "STATA software version 14.0 (Stata Corporation, College Station, TX, USA)," taking the multi-stage study sampling design into account (36). The sample was described with frequency distributions. Multinomial logistic regression was used to assess predictors of undiagnosed T2D and diagnosed T2D (versus no T2D). Logistic regressions were used to assess factors associated with undiagnosed T2D (versus diagnosed T2D). Variables significant in univariable analyses were included in the multivariable models. P-values <0.05 were considered significant.

Findings

The sample with complete fasting blood glucose measurement included 4,040 persons (18-69 years), with a mean age of 41.0 years (SD = 14.3 years) in 2018. The prevalence of undiagnosed T2D was 3.7% (3.6% of total T2D), diagnosed T2D 6.7%, and total T2D 10.4% (see Table 1).

Associations with undiagnosed and diagnosed T2D versus no diabetes

In the adjusted multinomial logistic regression analysis, older age (50-69 years) (ARRR: 7.93, 95% CI: 3.49-18.04), obesity (ARRR: 1.90, 95% CI: 1.14-3.14), and elevated total cholesterol (ARRR: 2.05, 95% CI: 1.40-3.00) were positively associated with undiagnosed T2D versus no T2D. Older age (50-69 years) (ARRR: 5.70, 95% CI: 2.61-12.45), health care visit (ARRR: 3.12, 95% CI: 2.12-4.57), obesity (ARRR: 1.56, 95% CI: 1.02-2.40), hypertension (ARRR: 1.52, 95% CI: 1.11-2.08), and elevated total cholesterol (ARRR: 1.60, 95% CI: 1.18-2.18) were positively associated with diagnosed T2D (versus no T2D) (see Tables 2 and 3).

Table 1. Sample characteristics, Ecuador 2018

Variable	**Sample**	**No diabetes**	**Undiagnosed type 2 diabetes**	**Diagnosed type 2 diabetes**
N	**4040**	**3591**	**180**	**269**
	N (%)	%	%	%
All		89.6	3.7	6.7
Predisposing factors				
Age (years)				
18-29	1039 (29.6)	97.6	0.7	1.7
30-49	1771 (41.0)	89.5	3.9	6.6
50-69	1230 (29.4)	81.6	6.4	12.0
Gender				
Female	2367 (51.6)	89.8	3.6	6.6
Male	1673 (48.4)	89.3	3.8	6.8
Marital status				
Not married	1823 (41.9)	91.0	3.4	5.6
Married	2212 (58.1)	88.5	3.9	7.5
Ethnicity				
Mestizo	3138 (79.5)	89.6	3.6	6.8
Amerindian	269 (5.6)	93.1	3.4	3.5
Montubio	321 (7.6)	87.0	4.3	8.6
African-Ecuadorian/Mulato	197 (4.2)	87.6	4.8	7.6
Whites/other	113 (3.1)	90.3	3.8	5.9
Enabling/disabling factors				
Health care visit (past 12 months)				
No	1663 (41.1)	93.0	4.0	3.0
Yes	2377 (58.9)	87.2	3.5	9.4

Table 1. (Continued)

Variable	Sample	No diabetes	Undiagnosed type 2 diabetes	Diagnosed type 2 diabetes
N	**4040**	**3591**	**180**	**269**
	N (%)	%	%	%
Formal education				
Less than secondary	2183 (48.9)	88.2	4.7	7.1
Secondary	815 (21.5)	90.0	2.9	7.1
More than Secondary	1038 (29.7)	91.5	2.5	6.0
Tobacco smoking				
Never	2644 (61.5)	90.4	3.5	6.1
Past	891 (24.7)	87.9	4.3	7.8
Current	505 (13.7)	88.9	3.5	7.6
Heavy alcohol use	871 (24.3)	89.8	4.3	5.9
Physical activity				
Low	948 (24.9)	87.7	4.4	7.9
Moderate	1062 (26.0)	89.1	3.8	7.2
High	2025 (49.2)	90.8	3.2	6.0
Need factors				
Body mass index				
Underweight	53 (1.7)	96.8	3.2	0.0
Normal	1313 (34.6)	92.9	2.2	4.9
Overweight	1536 (38.3)	91.1	3.3	5.6
Obesity	1064 (25.5)	82.4	6.1	11.5
Hypertension	836 (20.6)	82.4	5.1	12.5
Heart attack or stroke	366 (9.0)	88.4	3.9	7.6
Elevated total cholesterol	1186 (27.4)	82.4	6.8	10.8

Table 2. Unadjusted associations with undiagnosed and diagnosed type 2 diabetes (T2D)

Variable	Undiagnosed T2D Unadjusted RRR (95% CI)	Diagnosed T2D Unadjusted RRR (95% CI)
Predisposing factors		
Age (years)		
18-29	1 (Reference)	1 (Reference)
30-49	5.69 (2.82-11.49)***	4.28 (2.23-8.22)***
50-69	10.38 (5.03-21.40)***	8.50 (4.30-16.78)***
Gender		
Female	1 (Reference)	1 (Reference)
Male	1.08 (0.74-1.58)	1.04 (0.77-1.40)
Marital status		
Not married	1 (Reference)	1 (Reference)
Married	1.21 (0.82-1.78)	1.38 (1.02-1.86)*
Ethnicity		
Mestizo	1 (Reference)	1 (Reference)
Amerindian	0.92 (0.43-1.97)	0.49 (0.16-1.51)
Montubio	1.24 (0.57-2.71)	1.31 (0.80-2.14)
African-Ecuadorian/Mulato	1.38 (0.69-2.75)	1.14 (0.58-2.22)
Whites/other	1.04 (0.37-2.91)	0.87 (0.32-2.39)
Enabling/disabling factors		
Health care visit (past 12 months)		
No	1 (Reference)	1 (Reference)
Yes	0.91 (0.61-1.36)	3.35 (2.30-4.88)***
Formal education		
Less than secondary	1 (Reference)	1 (Reference)
Secondary	0.61 (0.36-1.01)	0.99 (0.64-1.52)
More than secondary	0.51 (0.30-0.87)*	0.82 (0.57-1.17)
Tobacco smoking		
Never	1 (Reference)	1 (Reference)
Past	1.27 (0.81-1.97)	1.30 (0.92-1.84)
Current	1.01 (0.56-1.83)	1.26 (0.79-1.99)
Heavy alcohol use	1.22 (0.76-1.95)	0.83 (0.56-1.23)
Physical activity		
Low	1 (Reference)	1 (Reference)
Moderate	0.84 (0.52-1.35)	0.90 (0.59-1.36)
High	0.69 (0.44-1.09)	0.73 (0.52-1.04)
Need factors		
Body mass index		
<25 kg/m^2	1 (Reference)	1 (Reference)
Overweight	1.53 (0.92-2.55)	1.22 (0.84-1.77)
Obesity	3.13 (1.89-5.17)***	2.79 (1.87-4.15)***
Hypertension	1.73 (1.15-2.62)**	2.62 (1.95-3.53)***
Heart attack or stroke	1.08 (0.57-2.06)	1.16 (0.74-1.81)
Elevated total cholesterol	3.02 (2.09-4.38)***	2.32 (1.73-3.12)***

RRR = Relative Risk Ratio; CI = Confidence Intervals; $*p < 0.05$; $**p < 0.01$; $***p < 0.001$.

Table 3. Adjusted associations with undiagnosed and diagnosed type 2 diabetes (T2D)

Variable	Undiagnosed T2D Adjusted RRR (95% CI)	Diagnosed T2D Adjusted RRR (95% CI)
Predisposing factors		
Age (years)		
18-29	1 (Reference)	1 (Reference)
30-49	4.63 (2.10-10.22)***	3.43 (1.62-7.25)***
50-69	7.93 (3.49-18.04)***	5.70 (2.61-12.45)***
Marital status		
Not married	1 (Reference)	1 (Reference)
Married	0.84 (0.56-1.24)	1.00 (0.71-1.40)
Enabling/disabling factors		
Health care visit (past 12 months)		
No	1 (Reference)	1 (Reference)
Yes	0.84 (0.55-1.28)	3.12 (2.12-4.57)***
Formal education		
Less than secondary	1 (Reference)	1 (Reference)
Secondary	0.81 (0.47-1.42)	1.25 (0.78-1.99)
More than secondary	0.81 (0.47-1.41)	1.06 (0.72-1.57)
Need factors		
Body mass index		
<25 kg/m^2	1 (Reference)	1 (Reference)
Overweight	1.04 (0.61-1.75)	0.81 (0.54-1.22)
Obesity	1.90 (1.14-3.14)*	1.56 (1.02-2.40)*
Hypertension	0.91 (0.61-1.36)	1.52 (1.11-2.08)**
Elevated total cholesterol	2.05 (1.40-3.00)***	1.60 (1.18-2.18)**

RRR = Relative Risk Ratio; CI = Confidence Intervals; *$p < 0.05$; **$p < 0.01$; ***$p < 0.001$.

Results of the binary logistic regression with undiagnosed T2D versus diagnosed T2D

In logistic regression analysis, only health care visit (AOR: 0.27, 95% CI: 0.16-0.47) was negatively associated with undiagnosed T2D (versus diagnosed T2D) (see Table 4).

Table 4. Associations with undiagnosed versus diagnosed type 2 diabetes

Variable	Unadjusted OR (95% CI)
Predisposing factors	
Age (years)	
18-29	1 (Reference)
30-49	1.33 (0.55-3.21)
50-69	1.22 (0.49-3.02)
Gender	
Female	1 (Reference)
Male	1.05 (0.66-1.66)
Marital status	
Not married	1 (Reference)
Married	0.88 (0.55-1.40)
Ethnicity	
Mestizo	1 (Reference)
Amerindian	1.86 (0.51-6.86)
Montubio	0.94 (0.40-2.24)
African-Ecuadorian/Mulato	1.21 (0.47-3.13)
Whites/other	1.20 (0.30-4.74)
Enabling/disabling factors	
Health care visit (past 12 months)	
No	1 (Reference)
Yes	0.27 (0.16-0.47)***
Formal education	
Less than secondary	1 (Reference)
Secondary	0.62 (0.32-1.20)
More than secondary	0.63 (0.32-1.21)
Tobacco smoking	
Never	1 (Reference)
Past	0.98 (0.56-1.71)
Current	0.80 (0.38-1.67)
Heavy alcohol use	1.46 (0.79-2.69)
Physical activity	
Low	1 (Reference)
Moderate	0.93 (0.51-1.70)
High	0.94 (0.54-1.62)
Need factors	
Body mass index	
<25 kg/m^2	1 (Reference)
Overweight	1.26 (0.67-2.35)
Obesity	1.12 (0.61-2.08)
Hypertension	0.66 (0.40-1.08)
Heart attack or stroke	0.93 (0.44-1.99)
Elevated total cholesterol	1.30 (0.82-2.07)

OR = Odds Ratio; CI = Confidence Intervals; ***$p < 0.001$.

Discussion

The study found a national prevalence of undiagnosed T2D (3.7%, 35.6% of total T2D), which is lower than recent global figures (44.7%) (6) and lower than in an earlier review of studies in 29 LMICs (4.9%) (7), lower than in a local study in Ecuador (11.6%) (10), and lower than in Suriname (39.6%) (8), lower than in China (6.9%, 63.3% of total T2D) (11), but higher than in northern Sudan (29.0%) (9).

In agreement with some research (13, 16-20, 24), we found that older age was associated with undiagnosed T2D (versus no T2D). In line with previous studies (12, 17, 30), enabling factors associated with undiagnosed T2D versus diagnosed T2D included no recent health care visit. People who use health care services may have reduced odds of undiagnosed T2D (13). Following the guidelines for the management of T2D in Ecuador, diabetic patients are expected to attend health care services more often (40), which may explain why people with diagnosed T2D visit health care providers more often than people with undiagnosed T2D (17). Previous studies (16, 21, 28) found mixed results regarding the association between educational status and undiagnosed T2D, while we found no significant association.

In agreement with previous research (18-20, 25, 26, 31-34), need factors associated with undiagnosed T2D included high total cholesterol and obesity. Unlike some previous studies (26, 31-34), we did not find an association between elevated total cholesterol, hypertension and undiagnosed T2D versus diagnosed T2D. The Ecuador national NCD programme includes local awareness campaigns on diabetes, early detection through basic health teams in the community, and integrated care for diabetes (41).

Study limitations include the cross-sectional study design and some data were assessed by self-report. Future studies may include additional measures, such as a family history of T2D and knowledge of symptoms of T2D.

Conclusion

A significant proportion of adults in Ecuador had undiagnosed T2D. Predisposing factors (older age), and need factors (high total cholesterol and obesity) were identified as associated with undiagnosed T2D (versus no T2D) and enabling factors (no recent health care visit) were identified as associated with undiagnosed T2D (versus diagnosed T2D).

Acknowledgments

This paper uses data from the 2018 Ecuador STEPS survey, implemented by the Ministry of Health with the support of the World Health Organization.

References

[1] World Health Organization. Diabetes factsheet, 2021. URL: https://www.who.int/news-room/fact-sheets/detail/diabetes.

[2] Fowler M. Microvascular and macrovascular complications of diabetes. Clin Diabetes 2011;29: 116–122.

[3] Vinik A, Flemmer M. Diabetes and macrovascular disease. J Diabetes Complicat 2002;16:235–45.

[4] Wild SH, Smith FB, Lee AJ, Fowkes FG. Criteria for previously undiagnosed diabetes and risk of mortality: 15-year follow-up of the Edinburgh Artery Study cohort. Diabetes Med 2005;22(4):490-6. doi: 10.1111/j.1464-5491.2004.01433.x.

[5] Valdés S, Botas P, Delgado E, Díaz Cadórniga F. Mortality risk in Spanish adults with diagnosed diabetes, undiagnosed diabetes or pre-diabetes. The Asturias study 1998-2004. Rev Esp Cardiol 2009;62(5):528-34. doi: 10.1016/s1885-5857(09)71835-3.

[6] Ogurtsova K, Guariguata L, Barengo NC, Ruiz PL, Sacre JW, et al. IDF diabetes atlas: Global estimates of undiagnosed diabetes in adults for 2021. Diabetes Res Clin Pract 2022;183:109118. doi: 10.1016/j.diabres.2021.109118.

[7] Seiglie JA, Marcus ME, Ebert C, Prodromidis N, Geldsetzer P, Theilmann M, et al. Diabetes prevalence and its relationship with education, wealth, and BMI in 29 low- and middle-income countries. Diabetes Care 2020;43(4):767-75. doi: 10.2337/dc19-1782.

[8] Krishnadath IS, Nahar-van Venrooij LM, Jaddoe VW, Toelsie JR. Ethnic differences in prediabetes and diabetes in the Suriname Health Study. BMJ Open Diabetes Res Care 2016;4(1):e000186. doi: 10.1136/bmjdrc-2015-000186.

[9] Eltom MA, Babiker Mohamed AH, Elrayah-Eliadarous H, Yassin K, Noor SK, et al. Increasing prevalence of type 2 diabetes mellitus and impact of ethnicity in north Sudan. Diabetes Res Clin Pract 2018;136:93-9. doi: 10.1016/j.diabres.2017.11.034.

[10] Tufton N, Chowdhury T. Prevalence of diabetes on Santa Cruz Island in Galapagos Archipelago. Prev Chronic Dis 2015;12:E94. doi: 10.5888/pcd12.150108.

[11] Wang L, Gao P, Zhang M, Huang Z, Zhang D, Deng Q, et al. Prevalence and ethnic pattern of diabetes and prediabetes in China in 2013. JAMA 2017;317(24):2515-23. doi: 10.1001/jama.2017.7596.

[12] Escobedo J, Buitrón LV, Velasco MF, Ramírez JC, Hernández R, Macchia A, et al. High prevalence of diabetes and impaired fasting glucose in urban Latin America: The CARMELA Study. Diabet Med 2009;26(9):864-71. doi: 10.1111/j.1464-5491.2009.02795.x.

[13] Andersen R. Revisiting the behavioral model and access to medical care: does it matter? J Health Soc Behav 1995;36(1):1–10. doi:10.2307/2137284.

[14] Mou C, Xu M, Lyu J. Predictors of undiagnosed diabetes among middle-aged and seniors in China: Application of Andersen's Behavioral Model. Int J Environ Res Public Health 2021;18(16):8396. doi: 10.3390/ijerph18168396.

[15] Lee S, Washburn DJ, Colwell B, Gwarzo IH, Kellstedt D, Ahenda P, et al. Examining social determinants of undiagnosed diabetes in Namibia and South Africa using a behavioral model of health services use. Diabetes Res Clin Pract 2021;175:108814. doi: 10.1016/j.diabres.2021.108814.

[16] Claypool KT, Chung MK, Deonarine A, Gregg EW, Patel CJ. Characteristics of undiagnosed diabetes in men and women under the age of 50 years in the Indian subcontinent: the National Family Health Survey (NFHS-4)/Demographic Health Survey 2015-2016. BMJ Open Diabetes Res Care 2020;8(1):e000965. doi: 10.1136/bmjdrc-2019-000965.

[17] Du Y, Baumert J, Paprott R, Teti A, Heidemann C, Scheidt-Nave C. Factors associated with undiagnosed type 2 diabetes in Germany: results from German Health Interview and Examination Survey for Adults 2008-2011. BMJ Open Diabetes Res Care 2020;8(1):e001707. doi: 10.1136/bmjdrc-2020-001707.

[18] Islam RM, Magliano DJ, Khan MN, Hossain MB, Rana J, Oldroyd JC. Prevalence of undiagnosed diabetes and the relative importance of its risk factors among adults in Bangladesh: Findings from a nationwide survey. Diabetes Res Clin Pract 2022;185:109228. doi: 10.1016/j.diabres.2022.109228.

[19] Heltberg A, Andersen JS, Sandholdt H, Siersma V, Kragstrup J, Ellervik C. Predictors of undiagnosed prevalent type 2 diabetes - The Danish General Suburban Population Study. Prim Care Diabetes 2018;12(1):13-22. doi: 10.1016/j.pcd. 2017.08.005.

[20] Mohammad A, Ziyab AH, Mohammad T. Prevalence of prediabetes and undiagnosed diabetes among Kuwaiti adults: A cross-sectional study. Diabetes Metab Syndr Obes 2021;14:2167-76. doi: 10.2147/DMSO.S296848.

[21] Hasan MM, Tasnim F, Tariqujjaman M, Ahmed S. Socioeconomic inequalities of undiagnosed diabetes in a resource-poor setting: Insights from the cross-sectional Bangladesh demographic and health survey 2011. Int J Environ Res Public Health 2019;16(1):115. doi: 10.3390/ijerph16010115.

[22] Heianza Y, Arase Y, Kodama S, Hsieh SD, Tsuji H, Saito K, et al. Association of living alone with the presence of undiagnosed diabetes in Japanese men: The role of modifiable risk factors for diabetes: Toranomon Hospital Health Management Center Study 13 (TOPICS 13). Diabetes Med 2013;30(11):1355-9. doi: 10.1111/dme.12255.

[23] Hsueh L, Wu W, Hirsh AT, de Groot M, Mather KJ, Stewart JC. Undiagnosed diabetes among immigrant and racial/ethnic minority adults in the United States: National Health and Nutrition Examination Survey 2011-2018. Ann Epidemiol 2020;51:14-9. doi: 10.1016/j.annepidem.2020.07.009.

[24] Coppell KJ, Mann JI, Williams SM, Jo E, Drury PL, Miller JC, et al. Prevalence of diagnosed and undiagnosed diabetes and prediabetes in New Zealand: Findings from the 2008/09 Adult Nutrition Survey. NZ Med J 2013126(1370):23-42.

[25] Bantie GM, Wondaye AA, Arike EB, Melaku MT, Ejigu ST, Lule A, et al. Prevalence of undiagnosed diabetes mellitus and associated factors among adult residents of Bahir Dar city, northwest Ethiopia: a community-based cross-sectional study. BMJ Open 2019;9(10):e030158. doi: 10.1136/bmjopen-2019-030158.

[26] O Connor JM, Millar SR, Buckley CM, Kearney PM, Perry IJ. The prevalence and determinants of undiagnosed and diagnosed type 2 diabetes in middle-aged Irish adults. PLoS One 2013;8(11):e80504. doi: 10.1371/journal.pone.0080504.

[27] Walker RJ, Garacci E, Ozieh M, Egede LE. Food insecurity and glycemic control in individuals with diagnosed and undiagnosed diabetes in the United States. Prim Care Diabetes 2021;15(5):813-8. doi: 10.1016/j.pcd.2021.05.003.

[28] Ruiz PL, Hopstock LA, Eggen AE, Njølstad I, Grimnes G, Stene LC, et al. Undiagnosed diabetes based on HbA_{1c} by socioeconomic status and healthcare consumption in the Tromsø Study 1994-2016. BMJ Open Diabetes Res Care 2021;9(2):e002423. doi: 10.1136/bmjdrc-2021-002423.

[29] Leahy S, O' Halloran AM, O' Leary N, Healy M, McCormack M, Kenny RA, et al. Prevalence and correlates of diagnosed and undiagnosed type 2 diabetes mellitus and pre-diabetes in older adults: Findings from the Irish Longitudinal Study on Ageing (TILDA). Diabetes Res Clin Pract 2015;110(3):241-9. doi: 10.1016/j.diabres.2015.10.015.

[30] Echouffo-Tcheugui JB, Dzudie A, Epacka ME, Choukem SP, Doualla MS, Luma H, et al. Prevalence and determinants of undiagnosed diabetes in an urban sub-Saharan African population. Prim Care Diabetes 2012;6(3):229-34. doi: 10.1016/j.pcd.2012.05.002.

[31] Pramono LA, Setiati S, Soewondo P, Subekti I, Adisasmita A, Kodim N, et al. Prevalence and predictors of undiagnosed diabetes mellitus in Indonesia. Acta Med Indones 2010;42(4):216-23.

[32] Nguyen VD, Vien QM, Do TH, Phan CD, Nguyen HC, Nguyen VT, et al. Prevalence of undiagnosed diabetes and pre-diabetes and its associated risk factors in Vietnam. J Glob Health Sci 2019;1(1):e7. https://doi.org/10.35500/jghs.2019.1.e7.

[33] Bjarkø VV, Haug EB, Sørgjerd EP, Stene LC, Ruiz PL, Birkeland KI, et al. Undiagnosed diabetes: Prevalence and cardiovascular risk profile in a population-based study of 52,856 individuals. The HUNT Study, Norway. Diabet Med 2022:e14829. doi: 10.1111/dme.14829.

[34] Apidechkul T, Chomchoei C, Upala P. Epidemiology of undiagnosed type 2 diabetes mellitus among hill tribe adults in Thailand. Sci Rep 2022;12(1):3969. doi: 10.1038/s41598-022-07977-9.

[35] World Health Organization. STEPwise approach to surveillance (STEPS), 2018. URL: https://www.who.int/ncds/surveillance/steps/en/ .

[36] Subsecretaría Nacional de Vigilancia de la Salud Pública, Subsecretaría Nacional de Promoción de la Salud e Igualdad, Dirección Nacional de Estrategias de Prevención y Control, Dirección Nacional de Promoción de la Salud (MSP, INEC, OPS/OMS). Encuesta STEPS Ecuador 2018. URL: https://extranet.who.int/ncdsmicrodata/index.php/catalog/774.

[37] Armstrong T, Bull F. Development of the World Health Organization Global Physical Activity Questionnaire (GPAQ). J Public Health 2006;14:66–70.

[38] Chobanian AV, Bakris GL, Black HR, Cushman WC, Green LA, Izzo JL et al. Seventh report of the Joint National Committee of Prevention, Detection, Evaluation, and Treatment of High Blood Pressure. Hypertension 2003;42(6):1206–52. http://dx.doi.org/10.1161/01.HYP.0000107251.49515.c2

[39] Expert Panel on Detection, Evaluation, and Treatment of High Blood Cholesterol in Adults. Executive Summary of the Third Report of The National Cholesterol Education Program (NCEP) Expert Panel on Detection, Evaluation, and Treatment of High Blood Cholesterol in Adults (Adult Treatment Panel III). JAMA 2001;285(19):2486-97. doi: 10.1001/jama.285.19.2486.

[40] Ministerio de Salud Pública del Ecuador. Diabetes mellitus tipo 2. Guía de Práctica Clínica. Quito: Ministerio de Salud Pública, Dirección Nacional de Normatización; 2017. URL: https://www.salud.gob.ec/wp-content/uploads/downloads/2017/05/Diabetes-mellitus_GPC.pdf.

[41] Dirección general de salud dirección de normatización del sistema nacional de salud dirección de control y mejoramiento de la salud pública. Plan estratégico nacional para la prevención y control de las enfermedades crónicas no transmisibles-ecnt, Ecuador, 2011. URL: https://www.iccp-portal.org/system/files/plans/ECU_B3_plan_estrategico_nacional_msp_final..pdf.

Chapter 15

Predictors of undiagnosed, diagnosed and total hypertension among adults in Afghanistan

Ahmad Siyar Noormal[1], MD, MSc, PhD
and Karl Peltzer[2,3,*], PhD

[1]Heidelberg Institute of Global Health, Heidelberg University, Heidelberg, Germany
[2]Department of Psychology, University of the Free State, Bloemfontein, South Africa
[3]Department of Psychology, College of Medical and Health Science, Asia University, Taichung, Taiwan

Abstract

In this chapter we aim to assess the prevalence and correlates of undiagnosed, diagnosed and total hypertension (HT) among adults in Afghanistan. The study analyzed cross-sectional national survey data from adults (N = 3,739, 18-69 years) in 2018. Results indicated that the prevalence of undiagnosed HT was 13.1% (36.9% of total HT), diagnosed HT 22.4%, and total HT 35.5%. Older age, high total cholesterol, and obesity were associated with undiagnosed HT (versus no HT), and male sex, never cholesterol measured, no obesity and no heart disease were associated with undiagnosed HT (versus diagnosed HT). Undiagnosed HT is common among adults in Afghanistan, calling for population-based interventions.

---

* ***Correspondence:*** Karl Peltzer, Department of Psychology, College of Medical and Health Sciences, Asia University, Wufeng, Taichung 41354, Taiwan.
Email: kfpeltzer@gmail.com.

In: Non-Communicable Diseases
Editor: Joav Merrick
ISBN: 979-8-89113-514-7

Introduction

Hypertension (HT) is a major cause of death globally and has been significantly increasing in developing countries (1-3), yet "only 1 in 3 are aware of their HT status." (3). If HT remains undiagnosed, treatment cannot be initiated which can lead to serious morbidity and mortality (4, 5). In Peru, 67.2% of people with HT had not been diagnosed (6). Among urban Chinese adults (20-79 years) 12.3% had undiagnosed HT and among hypertensives 37.3% (7). In Malaysia, among hypertensives 51.6% had undiagnosed HT (8), in Indonesia (≥40 years) 56.2% (9), and in Brunei Darussalam 28.6% had undiagnosed HT of total HT (10). In India among women (15-49 years) the prevalence of undiagnosed HT was 18.7% (11), among hypertensives in Bangladesh 50.1% were undiagnosed (5) and in Nepal 56.9% were undiagnosed (12). In 44 LMICs, 60.8% had undiagnosed HT of total HT (13). A study conducted in 2013 in Jalalabad city, Afghanistan found a prevalence of HT of 28.4%, and only 4% of hypertensive participants were previously diagnosed or were under treatment for HT (14). There are no national data on the prevalence and correlates of undiagnosed, diagnosed, and total hypertension (HT) among adults in Afghanistan, which led to the study.

Predisposing, enabling and need factors can be associated with undiagnosed HT (15, 16), including sociodemographic factors (5-8, 12, 17-19), socioeconomic status (5, 7-9, 11, 12, 18), geographic location (8, 11, 12, 18), health care utilisation (20), health insurance (6, 21), health behaviour (7, 8, 10, 22, 23), and chronic conditions (5-8, 11, 17, 19, 20, 24). The aim of the study was to assess the prevalence and correlates of undiagnosed, diagnosed and total HT among adults in Afghanistan.

Our study

We analysed national cross-sectional data from the 2018 Afghanistan STEPS survey (25), and restricted our sample to those with complete blood pressure measurement and non-pregnant (26). More details are published in (26). The 'Public Health Ministry of Afghanistan' ethics board approved the study and the participants gave their informed consent in writing.

Data collection followed the "WHO STEPS methodology: step 1 included administration of a structured questionnaire (sociodemographics, medical history, medication use, and health risk behaviours), step 2 consisted of blood pressure and anthropometric measurements, and step 3 included biochemical tests (blood glucose and blood lipids)." (26).

Measures

Undiagnosed HTN was defined as "systolic BP ≥140 mmHg and/or diastolic BP ≥90 mmHg among people who responded no the question, Have you ever been told by a doctor or other health worker that you have raised blood pressure or hypertension?" (6, 26, 27).

"Prior to taking blood pressure measurements, participants were asked to sit quietly and rest for 15 min with legs uncrossed. Three readings of systolic and diastolic blood pressure were obtained, with participants resting for three minutes between each reading. Of the three blood pressure measurements using the Omron BP apparatus automatic blood pressure monitor; the last two readings following recommendations by WHO were averaged" (26).

Sociodemographic (predisposing) factors included marital status, sex, age, and interview language (25).

Enhancing factors or barriers included educational level, cholesterol screening, education, economic status (adult household members), tobacco use, and physical activity levels (28).

Need factors consisted of diabetes, Body Mass Index (BMI), and elevated total cholesterol. BMI was classified as "underweight (<18.5 kg/m^2), normal weight (18.5-24.9 kg/m^2), overweight (25.0-29.9 kg/m^2), and obese (≥30.0 kg/m^2)" (26). *Diabetes:* "fasting plasma glucose levels >=7.0 mmol/L (≥126 mg/dl); or using insulin or oral hypoglycemic drugs" (26). Elevated total cholesterol: "being on antilipidemic medication or having elevated total cholesterol (TC) ≥190 mg/dl)" (25) History of heart attack or stroke was recorded if the respondent had answered positively to the question "Have you ever had a heart attack or chest pain from heart disease (angina) or a stroke (cerebrovascular accident or incident)? (Yes, No)" (26).

Analysis

Frequency distributions were calculated to describe the sample. Binary logistic regression was used to determine predictors of undiagnosed HT (versus diagnosed HT), and multinomial logistic regression with undiagnosed TH and diagnosed HT (versus no HT). P-values <0.05 were considered significant. Variables significant in univariable analyses were included in the multivariable models. Statistical analyses were done with "STATA software version 14.0 (Stata Corporation, College Station, TX, USA)," considering the multi-stage sampling design.

Findings

The final sample included 3,739 persons (18-69 years, median age 36 years, IQR: 25-49 years). The prevalence of undiagnosed HT was 13.1% (36.9% of total HT), diagnosed HT was 22.4% and total HT 35.5% (see Table 1).

Multinomial logistic regression results

In the adjusted multinomial logistic regression analysis, older age (45-69 years) (Adjusted Relative Risk Ratio-ARRR: 2.23, 95% CI: 1.40-4.54), obesity (ARRR: 3.86, 95% CI: 2.34-6.37), and elevated total cholesterol (ARRR: 2.33, 95% CI: 1.56-3.49) were positively associated with undiagnosed HT versus no HT. Older age (45-69 years) (ARRR: 2.87, 95% CI: 1.57-5.24), ever cholesterol screening (ARRR: 6.40, 95% CI: 4.20-9.77), obesity (ARRR: 2.13, 95% CI: 1.48-3.05), and heart attack or stroke (ARRR: 3.13, 95% CI: 1.76-5.58), were positively associated, and male sex (ARRR: 0.64, 95% CI: 0.29-0.75) and higher education (ARRR: 0.47, 95% CI: 0.24-0.94) were negatively associated with diagnosed HT versus no HT (see Tables 2 and 3).

Results of binary logistic regression

In adjusted logistic regression analysis, male sex (AOR: 2.33, 95% CI: 1.27-4.29) increased odds and ever measured cholesterol (AOR: 0.18, 95% CI: 0.10-0.33), and heart attack or stroke (AOR: 0.34, 95% CI: 0.16-0.74) decreased odds of undiagnosed HT (versus diagnosed HT) (see Table 4).

Table 1. Sample characteristics, Afghanistan 2018

Variable	Sample	No hypertension	Undiagnosed hypertension	Diagnosed hypertension
N	**3739**	**2359**	**560**	**820**
	N (%)	%	%	%
All		64.5	13.1	22.4
Predisposing factors				
Age (years)				
18-29	1355 (43.7)	74.9	9.6	15.6
30-44	1118 (32.5)	65.2	13.2	21.7
45-69	1240 (23.9)	44.7	19.3	36.0
Gender				
Female	1734 (44.0)	57.5	11.9	30.6
Male	2005 (56.0)	70.0	14.0	16.0
Marital status				
Not married	767 (25.2)	76.1	8.7	15.2
Married	2971 (74.8)	60.6	14.6	24.9
Enabling/disabling factors				
Residence				
Rural	1775 (42.3)	64.2	11.9	23.8
Urban	1964 (57.7)	64.7	13.9	21.4
Number of adult household members				
<5	1971 (39.4)	61.8	15.3	22.9
≥5	1768 (60.6)	66.3	11.7	22.1
Education in years				
None	2080 (59.0)	58.1	13.6	28.2
≤Primary	650 (16.4)	64.1	15.9	20.0
≥Secondary	1009 (24.6)	80.0	9.8	10.2

Table 1. (Continued)

Variable	Sample	No hypertension	Undiagnosed hypertension	Diagnosed hypertension
N	**3739**	**2359**	**560**	**820**
	N (%)	%	%	%
Ever cholesterol screening				
No	3101 (81.0)	71.2	14.0	14.8
Yes	638 (19.0)	35.9	8.9	55.2
Current tobacco use	860 (28.2)	62.6	14.3	23.0
Physical activity				
Low	1365 (38.2)	57.6	13.2	29.2
Moderate	621 (18.5)	63.2	13.0	23.8
High	1721 (43.3)	71.1	13.0	15.8
Need factors				
Body mass index				
Normal	1767 (49.4)	74.1	9.5	16.4
Underweight	264 (7.8)	88.2	3.3	8.5
Overweight	1071 (25.6)	55.1	18.0	26.8
Obesity	635 (17.2)	39.9	20.5	39.6
Diabetes	403 (9.8)	36.9	18.9	44.2
Heart attack or stroke	286 (9.5)	41.1	9.1	49.8
Elevated total cholesterol	641 (16.8)	39.5	19.4	41.1

Table 2. Unadjusted associations with undiagnosed and diagnosed hypertension (versus no hypertension

Variable	**Undiagnosed hypertension**	**Diagnosed hypertension**
	Unadjusted RRR (95% CI)	**Unadjusted RRR (95% CI)**
Predisposing factors		
Age (years)		
18-29	1 (Reference)	1 (Reference)
30-44	1.58 (1.05-2.38)*	1.60 (0.97-2.64)
45-69	3.37 (2.22-5.13)***	3.88 (2.36-6.35)***
Gender		
Female	1 (Reference)	1 (Reference)
Male	0.97 (0.64-1.48)	0.43 (0.30-0.61)***
Marital status		
Not married	1 (Reference)	1 (Reference)
Married	2.11 (1.22-3.67)**	2.05 (1.20-3.52)**
Enabling/disabling factors		
Residence		
Rural	1 (Reference)	1 (Reference)
Urban	1.15 (0.72-1.86)	0.89 (0.59-1.35)
Number of adult household members		
<5	1 (Reference)	1 (Reference)
≥5	0.71 (0.44-1.14)	0.90 (0.57-1.42)
Education in years		
None	1 (Reference)	1 (Reference)
≤Primary	1.06 (0.68-1.65)	0.64 (0.41-1.00)
≥Secondary	0.52 (0.35-0.78)***	0.26 (0.15-0.46)***
Ever cholesterol screening		
No	1 (Reference)	1 (Reference)
Yes	1.25 (0.72-2.18)	7.41 (5.11-10.74)***
Current tobacco use	1.19 (0.81-1.73)	1.08 (0.68-1.73)
Physical activity		
Low	1 (Reference)	1 (Reference)
Moderate	0.89 (0.53-1.49)	0.74 (0.48-1.14)
High	0.80 (0.57-1.11)	0.44 (0.27-0.70)***
Need factors		
Body mass index		
<25 kg/m^2	1 (Reference)	1 (Reference)
Overweight	2.88 (1.93-4.28)***	2.42 (1.55-3.78)***
Obesity	4.52 (2.63-.7.77)***	4.93 (3.39-7.18)***
Diabetes	2.77 (1.16-6.63)*	3.91 (2.14-7.16)***
Heart attack or stroke	1.10 (0.44-2.77)	4.15 (2.09-8.26)***
Elevated total cholesterol	2.86 (1.96-4.16)***	3.80 (2.29-6.30)***

RRR = Relative Risk Ratio; CI = Confidence Intervals; *$p < 0.05$; **$p < 0.01$; ***$p < 0.001$.

Table 3. Adjusted associations with undiagnosed and diagnosed hypertension (versus no hypertension)

Variable	Undiagnosed hypertension	Diagnosed hypertension
	Adjusted RRR (95% CI)	**Adjusted RRR (95% CI)**
Predisposing factors		
Age (years)		
18-29	1 (Reference)	1 (Reference)
30-44	1.17 (0.74-1.84)	1.15 (0.61-2.18)
45-69	2.23 (1.40-3.54)***	2.87 (1.57-5.24)***
Gender		
Female	1 (Reference)	1 (Reference)
Male	1.25 (0.80-1.94)	0.46 (0.29-0.75)**
Marital status		
Not married	1 (Reference)	1 (Reference)
Married	1.11 (0.57-2.15)	1.31 (0.66-2.61)
Enabling/disabling factors		
Education in years		
None	1 (Reference)	1 (Reference)
≤Primary	1.33 (0.82-2.16)	1.24 (0.61-2.18)
≥Secondary	0.64 (0.39-1.05)	0.47 (0.24-0.94)*
Ever cholesterol screening		
No	1 (Reference)	1 (Reference)
Yes	0.90 (0.55-1.48)	6.40 (4.20-9.77)***
Physical activity		
Low	1 (Reference)	1 (Reference)
Moderate	0.96 (0.56-1.67)	0.95 (0.60-1.50)
High	0.92 (0.64-1.33)	0.71 (0.39-1.29)
Need factors		
Body mass index		
<25 kg/m^2	1 (Reference)	1 (Reference)
Overweight	2.37 (1.51-3.72)***	1.54 (0.94-2.52)
Obesity	3.86 (2.34-6.37)***	2.13 (1.48-3.05)***
Diabetes	1.53 (0.73-3.24)	1.48 (0.80-2.72)
Heart attack or stroke	0.88 (0.38-2.05)	3.13 (1.76-5.58)***
Elevated total cholesterol	2.33 (1.56-3.49)***	1.63 (0.97-2.74)

RRR = Relative Risk Ratio; CI = Confidence Intervals; *$p < 0.05$; **$p < 0.01$; *** $p < 0.001$.

Discussion

The prevalence of undiagnosed HT in Afghanistan (13.1%; 36.9% of total HT), was lower than in 44 LMICs (60.8% of HT) (13), a study in Jalalabad city, Afghanistan (25-65 years) in 2013 (96% of HT) (17), in Malaysia (51.6% of HT) (8), in Bangladesh (50.1% of HT) (5), in Nepal (56.9% of HT) (12), and in Peru (67.2% of HT) (6), similar to China (12.3%; 37.3% of HT) (7), and higher than Brunei Darussalam (28.6% of HT) (10). People in Afghanistan may generally lack of awareness of routine blood pressure screening (14).

Table 4. Associations with undiagnosed versus diagnosed hypertension

Variable	**Unadjusted OR (95% CI)**	**Adjusted OR (95% CI)**
Predisposing factors		
Age (years)		
18-29	1 (Reference)	---
30-44	0.99 (0.58-1.67)	
45-69	0.87 (0.56-1.36)	
Gender		
Female	1 (Reference)	1 (Reference)
Male	2.27 (1.50-3.44)***	2.33 (1.27-4.29)**
Marital status		
Not married	1 (Reference)	---
Married	1.03 (0.56-1.89)	
Enabling/disabling factors		
Residence		
Rural	1 (Reference)	---
Urban	1.30 (0.72-2.32)	
Number of adult household members		
<5	1 (Reference)	---
≥5	0.79 (0.45-1.40)	
Education in years		
None	1 (Reference)	1 (Reference)
≤Primary	1.65 (0.90-3.02)	1.05 (0.48-2.33)
≥Secondary	1.99 (1.09-3.64)*	1.47 (0.63-3.43)
Ever cholesterol screening		
No	1 (Reference)	1 (Reference)
Yes	0.17 (0.09-0.31)***	0.18 (0.10-0.33)***
Current tobacco use	1.10 (0.70-1.71)	---
Physical activity		
Low	1 (Reference)	1 (Reference)
Moderate	1.20 (0.69-2.09)	1.14 (0.59-2.19)
High	1.81 (1.11-2.97)*	1,23 (0.75-2.02)
Need factors		
Body mass index		
<25 kg/m^2	1 (Reference)	---
Overweight	1.19 (0.79-1.79)	
Obesity	0.92 (0.51-1.66)	
Diabetes	0.71 (0.32-1.57)	---
Heart attack or stroke	0.27 (0.12-0.57)***	0.34 (0.16-0.74)**
Elevated total cholesterol	0.75 (0.48-1.18)	---

OR = Odds Ratio; CI = Confidence Intervals; **p < 0.05; **p < 0.01; ***p < 0.001.*

We found that men, older persons and those who had not screened for cholesterol were more likely to have undiagnosed HT (versus no HT or diagnosed HT), which is consistent with former studies (5-8, 18, 20, 23). Men may less likely be diagnosed for HT because they may visit health facilities less frequently than women, so women have a higher chance of HT screening than men (10). Therefore, men, those that had not screened for cholesterol, and older persons should be targeted in HT screening programmes. Contrary to some previous research (8, 11), we did not find a significant association between rural residence, lower education and undiagnosed HT. Furthermore, we found an association between high total cholesterol, obesity but not diabetes, with undiagnosed HT. These results partially confirm previous results (7, 8, 11, 24) and document the contribution of obesity and high total cholesterol to HT (24).

The following policy implications are extracted from the study results: increased media campaigns on public awareness, community mobilization and education, targeting healthy body weight, cholesterol levels, HT screening and secondary HT prevention in Afghanistan (8, 14, 29). Study limitations include the cross-sectional nature of the study, and the evaluation of some variables by self-report.

Conclusion

Undiagnosed HT is common among adults in Afghanistan, calling for population-based HT screening targeting men, older persons, those that never screened for cholesterol, are obese and have high cholesterol levels.

Acknowledgments

This paper uses data from the 2018 Afghanistan STEPS survey, implemented by the Ministry of Public Health with the support of the World Health Organization.

References

[1] World Health Organization. Factsheet hypertension, 2021. URL: https://www.who.int/news-room/fact-sheets/detail/hypertension.

[2] NCD Risk Factor Collaboration (NCD-RisC). Worldwide trends in hypertension prevalence and progress in treatment and control from 1990 to 2019: a pooled analysis of 1201 population-representative studies with 104 million participants. Lancet 2021;398(10304):957-80. doi: 10.1016/S0140-6736(21)01330-1.

[3] Schutte AE, Srinivasapura Venkateshmurthy N, Mohan S, Prabhakaran D. Hypertension in low- and middle-income countries. Circ Res 2021;128(7):808-26. doi: 10.1161/CIRCRESAHA.120.318729.

[4] Lackland DT, Weber MA. Global burden of cardiovascular disease and stroke: hypertension at the core. Can J Cardiol 2015;31(5):569-71. doi: 10.1016/j.cjca.2015.01.009.

[5] Haider MR, Gupta RD. Inequalities in undiagnosed hypertension among adult population in Bangladesh: Evidence from a nationally representative survey. High Blood Press Cardiovasc Prev 2022;29(1):57-64. doi: 10.1007/s40292-021-00488-0.

[6] Guerrero-Díaz DV, Hernández-Vásquez A, Montoya-Rivera WC, Rojas-Roque C, Chacón Díaz MA, Bendezu-Quispe G. Undiagnosed hypertension in Peru: analysis of associated factors and socioeconomic inequalities, 2019. Heliyon 2021;7(7):e07516. doi: 10.1016/j.heliyon.2021.e07516.

[7] Zhang H, Deng M, Xu H, Wang H, Song F, Bao C, et al. Pre- and undiagnosed-hypertension in urban Chinese adults: a population-based cross-sectional study. J Hum Hypertens 2017;31(4):263-9. doi: 10.1038/jhh.2016.73.

[8] Lim OW, Yong CC. The risk factors for undiagnosed and known hypertension among Malaysians. Malays J Med Sci 2019;26(5):98-112. doi: 10.21315/mjms2019.26.5.9.

[9] Mahwati Y, Nurrika D, Latief K. The determinants of undiagnosed hypertension among Indonesian adults: A cross-sectional study based on the 2014-2015 Indonesia Family Life Survey. J Prev Med Public Health 2022;55(1):60-7. doi: 10.3961/jpmph.21.500.

[10] Ong SK, Kahan SZ, Lai DTC, Si-Ramlee KA, Abdullah MA, Nazurah Sidup N. et al. Prevalence of undetected hypertension and its association with socio-demographic and non-communicable diseases risk factors in Brunei Darussalam. J Public Health (Berlin) 2020 May 16. https://doi.org/10.1007/s10389-020-01287-y.

[11] Talukdar D, Tripathi M, Tripathi V, Teelucksingh S. Prevalence and associated factors of undiagnosed hypertension among women aged 15-49 years in India: an analysis of National Family Health Survey-4 data. J Hum Hypertens 2021;35(8):726-40. doi: 10.1038/s41371-020-0384-7.

[12] Haider MR, Das Gupta R. Inequalities in undiagnosed hypertension among adult Nepalese population: Evidence from a nationally representative survey. Int J Cardiol Hypertens 2020;5:100026. doi: 10.1016/j.ijchy.2020.100026.

[13] Geldsetzer P, Manne-Goehler J, Marcus ME, Ebert C, Zhumadilov Z, Wesseh CS, et al. The state of hypertension care in 44 low-income and middle-income countries: a cross-sectional study of nationally representative individual-level data from 1.1 million adults. Lancet 2019;394(10199):652-62. doi: 10.1016/S0140-6736(19)30955-9.

[14] Saeed KMI. Prevalence of hypertension and associated factors in Jalalabad City, Nangarhar Province, Afghanistan. Cent Asian J Glob Health 2015;4(1):134. doi: 10.5195/cajgh.2015.134.

[15] Andersen R. Revisiting the behavioral model and access to medical care: Does it matter? J Health Soc Behav 1995;36(1):1–10. doi:10.2307/2137284.

[16] Mou C, Xu M, Lyu J. Predictors of undiagnosed diabetes among middle-aged and seniors in China: Application of Andersen's Behavioral Model. Int J Environ Res Public Health 2021;18(16):8396. doi: 10.3390/ijerph18168396.

[17] Cham B, Scholes S, Ng Fat L, Badjie O, Mindell JS. Burden of hypertension in The Gambia: evidence from a national World Health Organization (WHO) STEP survey. Int J Epidemiol 2018;47(3):860-871. doi: 10.1093/ije/dyx279.

[18] Hasan MM, Tasnim F, Tariqujjaman M, Ahmed S, Cleary A, Mamun A. Examining the prevalence, correlates and inequalities of undiagnosed hypertension in Nepal: a population-based cross-sectional study. BMJ Open 2020;10(10):e037592. doi: 10.1136/bmjopen-2020-037592.

[19] Chau K, Girerd N, Zannad F, Rossignol P, Boivin JM. Health-related determinants of undiagnosed arterial hypertension: a population-based study. Fam Pract 2019;36(3):276-83. doi: 10.1093/fampra/cmy075.

[20] Zhou J, Fang S. Association between undiagnosed hypertension and health factors among middle-aged and elderly Chinese population. Int J Environ Res Public Health 2019;16(7):1214. doi: 10.3390/ijerph16071214.

[21] Morey BN, Valencia C, Lee S. Correlates of undiagnosed hypertension among Chinese and Korean American immigrants. J Commun Health 2022;47(3):425-36. doi: 10.1007/s10900-022-01069-5.

[22] Haligamo D, Ayalew A, Genemo H, Yiriga N. Undiagnosed hypertension and its associated factors among adult people living in Southern Ethiopia: Evidence from Gunchire Woreda of Gurage Zone. J Hypertens Manag 2021;7:063. doi.org/10.23937/2474-3690/1510063.

[23] Datta BK, Husain MJ. Uncontrolled hypertension among tobacco-users: women of prime childbearing age at risk in India. BMC Women's Health 2021;21:146. https://doi.org/10.1186/s12905-021-01280-x.

[24] Mogas SB, Tesfaye T, Zewde B, Tesfaye Y, Kebede A, Tadesse M, et al. Burden of undiagnosed hypertension among adults in urban communities of Southwest Ethiopia. Integr Blood Press Control 2021;14:69-76. doi: 10.2147/IBPC.S293251.

[25] World Health Organization. STEPwise approach to surveillance (STEPS), 2018. URL: https://www.who.int/ncds/surveillance/steps/en/.

[26] JS Consultancy Services. Non-communicable disease risk factor survey country report for Afghanistan. URL: https://extranet.who.int/ncdsmicrodata/index.php/catalog/782.

[27] Chobanian AV, Bakris GL, Black HR, Cushman WC, Green LA, Izzo JL et al. Seventh report of the Joint National Committee of Prevention, Detection, Evaluation, and Treatment of High Blood Pressure. Hypertension 2003;42(6):1206–52. http://dx.doi.org/10.1161/01.HYP.0000107251.49515.c2.

[28] Armstrong T, Bull F. Development of the World Health Organization Global Physical Activity Questionnaire (GPAQ). J Public Health 2006;14:66–70.

[29] Ministry of Public Health. Afghanistan General Directorate of Preventive Medicine Noncommunicable Diseases Control Directorate. National strategy for prevention and control of noncommunicable diseases (NCDs), 2015-2020. URL: https://extranet.who.int/ncdccs/Data/AFG_B3_National-NCD-Strategy-2015-2020-English2512201612411892755332532 5.pdf.

Chapter 16

Suicide attempt among school-based adolescents in Bolivia: Risk factors and gender differences

Lyen Krenz Yap[1], RPm, MSc
Karl Peltzer[1,2,*], PhD
Zuchi Lkhamsuren[1], MSc
and Passakorn Suanrueang[3], PhD
[1]Department of Psychology, College of Medical and Health Science, Asia University, Taiwan
[2]Department of Psychology, University of the Free State, Bloemfontein, South Africa
[3]Department of Healthcare Administration Specialty in Psychology, College of Medical and Health Science, Asia University, Taiwan

Abstract

In this chapter we investigate the risk factors and gender differences for suicide attempts among adolescents in Bolivia. This research involved a secondary analysis of the 2018 Bolivia cross-sectional Global School-Based Student Health Survey. The sample included 7,931 school adolescents (49.7% females and 50.3% males), and the mean age was 15.5 years (SD = 1.6) (age range = 11 years to = 18 years). In all, 21.4% of participants had attempted suicide in the last 12 months, 25.7% among females, and 17.5% among males. In adjusted logistic regression analysis, specifically among males, lifetime amphetamine use (AOR: 3.16, 95% CI: 1.28, 7.78), being physically attacked (AOR: 1.36, 95%

* ***Correspondence:*** Karl Peltzer, Department of Psychology, College of Medical and Health Science, Asia University, Wufeng, Taichung 41354, Taiwan; Email: kfpeltzer@gmail.com.

In: Non-Communicable Disease
Editor: Joav Merrick
ISBN: 979-8-89113-514-7

CI: 1.00, 1.84), bullied (AOR: 1.87, 95% CI: 1.51, 2.32), and experiencing psychological distress (AOR: 2.69, 95% CI: 2.04, 3.54) increased the odds of past 12-month suicide attempts. In adjusted logistic regression analysis, specifically among females, current alcohol use (AOR: 1.78, 95% CI: 1.30, 2.42), current cannabis use (AOR: 1.98, 95% CI: 1.06, 3.67), being physically attacked (AOR: 2.04, 95% CI: 1.46, 2.85), being in a physical fight (AOR: 1.61, 95% CI: 1.24, 2.10), injury (AOR: 1.38, 95% CI: 1.10, 1.75), and experiencing psychological distress (AOR: 3.02, 95% CI: 2.44, 3.73) increased the odds of past 12-month suicide attempts. More than one in five students (one in four females) had attempted suicide in the last 12 months in Bolivia. Several general and gender-specific factors were identified to increase the odds of suicide attempts, which can assist in designing suicide prevention in this adolescent population.

Introduction

Suicidal ideation is described as "thoughts or wishes to be dead or to kill oneself" whereas suicide attempts are "self-inflicted behaviors intended to result in death" (1). According to the World Health Organization (2) suicide takes about 700,000 people's lives every year, and among adolescents (15-19 years) suicide is the fourth leading cause of mortality globally. The World Health Organization (2) also estimates that 77% of suicides take place in countries with a struggling economy. The 12-month prevalence for suicide attempts among adolescents was 17.4% across low- to middle-income countries (3).

On the connection between negative health behaviors and suicide, literature in low- to middle-income countries shows that high levels of sedentary behavior (4), smoking, amphetamine use (5), cannabis use (6) and alcohol use (7) were prevalent in school-going adolescents who attempted suicide. Factors associated with suicidal behaviors among adolescents also include being physically attacked and physical fighting (4), loneliness (7), anxiety, having no close friends (4), and being bullied (5).

In Latin America, suicidal behaviors are the third leading cause of mortality among young people (8), with 65,000 suicides occurring among young people each year (9). In another cross-sectional study across countries in Latin America and the Caribbean, the prevalence of suicidal attempts in the past 12 months was 9.3% for male adolescents and higher for female adolescents at 16.3% (10). In an analysis of a combined Global School Health Surveys in Latin America, Bolivia in 2012 had the highest percentage of school-going adolescents who reported at least one suicide attempt (20.9%) and multiple suicide attempts (7.4%) in the past 12 months (11).

According to the World Bank, Bolivia is a lower middle-income country (12). It's heralded as one of poorest countries in Latin America suffering from both rural and urban poverty (13). Bolivia's universal healthcare system only came to existence in 2007, and it wasn't until 2009 that they launched a National Mental Health Plan in response to the lack of mental health policy, support and promotion (14).

In a review of the psychiatric situation in Bolivia by Jaen-Varas and colleagues (15), there are only 1.06 psychiatrists, 0.46 psychologists, and 0.25 social workers for every 100,000 members of the population. Suicide mortality rates are underreported, with suicide as the cause of death among 40% of the youths in Alto city and a reported rate of 430 suicides per 100,000 individuals in the community (16). Jørs and colleagues (17) set out to find information on suicidal behavior among adolescents, young adults, and older adults in Bolivia and found gender differences in suicide attempts and suicide, with more women (61%) attempting suicide than men, but more men (70.5%) committing suicide than women.

In Bolivia, specifically in La Paz, a study of the Youth Risk Behavior Survey (YRBS) among 13–18-year old's indicated gender differences in risk factors: females who were depressed, had low academic performance, experienced sexual abuse, and had increased alcoholic consumption were found to be more prone to suicide attempts whereas risk factors for men included being harassed on school property, including being threatened or injured (18).

While there have been some local studies on the prevalence and risk factors for suicide attempts among youth in Bolivia, this study hopes to fill the literature gap using the 2018 Global School Health Survey to provide a more recent report on the national situation. Moreover, this study provides a more comprehensive account by including gender differences.

Given Bolivia's economic instability and poor mental health situation, combined with the high vulnerability to suicide by the adolescent population, this study aims to investigate the risk factors and gender differences for suicide attempts among adolescents in Bolivia. Results of this study may have significant contributions to pertinent shareholders about the psychiatric situation in Bolivia as well as implications for potential target-oriented public health interventions.

Our study

This research involved a secondary analysis of the cross-sectional 2018 Bolivia Global School-Based Student Health Survey, which used a two-stage cluster sampling strategy to produce data characteristic of all students in 2nd Secondary - 6th Secondary in Bolivia (19). In the initial stage, schools were chosen based on probability proportional to enrollment size, and at the latter stage, random selection was applied to the classes, and students who were eligible to participate were selected (19). A total of 7,931 students participated with an overall response rate of 79% (19). Approval was granted by Bolivia's Ministry of Health along with a national ethics committee to proceed with the study protocol, and "necessary approvals and permits, including informed consent, were obtained from the participating schools, the parents, and the students before the survey was administered."

Measures

This study utilized the 2018 Global School Health Survey Questionnaire for Bolivia (19) for Bolivia, which comprised three major categories of risk factors: substance use, interpersonal violence and injury, and psychological distress. Table 1 describes the questionnaire items used in this study.

Dependent variable

Suicide attempt was assessed with the item "During the past 12 months, how many times did you actually attempt suicide?". Response options ranged from "0 times to 6 or more times," and coded 0 = 0 times and 1 = 1 to 6 or more times.

Covariates

Sociodemographic factors included sex and age group.

Risk factors

Substance use as a risk factor comprised of three variables: current alcohol use, current cannabis use, and lifetime amphetamine or methamphetamine use. Interpersonal violence and injury as a risk factor comprised of four variables: being physically attacked, physical fighting, injury, and being bullied. Table

1 describes the questionnaire items, response options, and coding scheme used for this study.

Psychological distress as a variable was measured with two items, assessing loneliness "During the past 12 months, how often have you felt lonely?" and "During the past 12 months, how often have you been so worried about something that you could not sleep at night?". There were five scales for response with codes as "Never = 0, Rarely = 1, Sometimes = 1, Most of the time = 2, Always = 3". Scores of the two items were added and scores resulting in three or higher were labelled as psychological distress. Cronbach alpha for the 2-item of psychological distress variables was 0.61.

Analysis of data

Data Interpretation was accomplished using STATA software version 15.1 (Stata Corporation, College Station, TX, USA), bearing in mind the multi-stage sampling design and weighting of the data. Initial descriptions of the data were reported using frequencies and percentages. Logistic regression was employed to identify factors associated with the outcome variable of suicide attempts (past 12 months), including differences between boys and girls. Variables significant in the unadjusted models were subsequently included in the adjusted model. Missing cases were omitted from the analysis. Significance was regarded at $P < 0.05$.

Findings

The sample included 7,931 school adolescents (50.3% males, and 49.7% females), and the mean age was 15.5 years (SD = 1.6) (age range =11 years to =18 years). Among the students, 26.4% were current alcohol users, 7.8% were current cannabis users, and 4.5% had ever used amphetamine. Furthermore, 28.6% have reported being physically attacked, 30.6% have been involved in physical fighting, 24.7% reported being bullied, and slightly more than half (52.1%) reported being seriously injured in the past year. 22.3% of the sample experienced psychological distress. In all, 21.4% of students had attempted suicide in the past 12 months, 25.7% among females, and 17.5% among males (see Table 2).

Table 1. Description of variables

Variable	Question	Response Options (Coding Scheme)
Age	"How old are you?"	"11 year old or younger to 18 years old or older" (Coded 1= 11 years old and younger to 14 years old, 2 = 15 years old, 3 = 16 years old, 4 = 17 years and older)
Sex	"What is your sex?"	"Male, Female" (Coded 0= Female, 1= Male)
Suicide Attempt	"During the past 12 months, how many times did you actually attempt suicide?"	"0 times to 6 or more times" (Coded 0 = 0 times, 1 = 1 to 6 or more times)
Risk Factors – Substance Use		
Current Alcohol Use	"During the past 30 days, on how many days did you have at least one drink containing alcohol?"	"0 days to All 30 Days" (Coded 0 = 0 days, 1 = 1 to 30 days)
Current Cannabis Use	"During the past 30 days, how many times have you used marijuana (also called maria juana, yerba, or mota)?"	"0 times to 20 or more times" (Coded 0 = 0 times, 1 = 1 to 20 or more times)
Amphetamine Use	"During your life, how many times have you used amphetamines or methamphetamines (also called pastillas or pepas)?"	"0 times to 20 or more times" (Coded 0 = 0 times, 1 = 1 to 20 or more times)
Risk Factors – Interpersonal violence and injury		
Physically Attacked	"During the past 12 months, how many times were you physically attacked?"	"0 times to 12 or more times" (Coded 0 = 0 times, 1= 1 to 12 or more times)
Physical Fighting	"During the past 12 months, how many times were you in a physical fight?"	"0 times to 12 or more times" (Coded 0 = 0 times, 1 = 1 to 12 or more times)
Bullied	"During the past 12 months, have you ever been bullied on school property?"	"Yes, No" (Coded 0 = No, 1 = Yes)
Injury	"During the past 12 months, how many times were you seriously injured?"	"0 times to 12 or more times" (Coded 0 = 0 times, 1 = 1 to 12 or more times)
Risk Factors – Psychological distress		
Loneliness	"During the past 12 months, how often have you felt lonely?"	"Never to Always" (Coded 0 = Never, 1 = Rarely, 2 = Sometimes, 3 = Most of the time, 4 = Always)
Anxiety	"During the past 12 months, how often have you been so worried about something that you could not sleep at night?"	"Never to Always" (Coded 0 = Never, 1 = Rarely, 2 = Sometimes, 3 = Most of the time, 4 = Always)

Table 2. Descriptive statistics, school adolescents in Bolivia, 2018

Variable (# missing cases)	**Total Sample**			**Suicide Attempt**		
	All N (%)	**Male N (%)**	**Female N (%)**	**All N (%)**	**Male N (%)**	Female N (%)
Socio-demographics	7,931			1,634 (21.4) #296		
Sex (#154)						
Male	4,014 (50.3)			665 (17.5)		
Female	3,763 (49.7)			918 (25.7)		
Age in Years (#95)						
≤11 to 14	2,366 (30.5)	1,142 (14.9)	1,170 (15.3)	509 (6.9)	187 (14.8)	302 (15.3)
15	1,593 (20.4)	764 (10.1)	813 (10.4)	324 (4.4)	145 (10.1)	172 (10.4)
16	1,591 (19.9)	772 (10.0)	800 (9.9)	316 (4.2)	122 (10.1)	185 (10.0)
17+	2,286 (29.3)	1064 (15.6)	1204 (13.8)	462 (6.3)	202 (15.6)	256 (13.7)
Risk Factors – Substance Use						
Current Alcohol Use (#474)	1,998 (26.4)	1,041 (13.9)	894 (12.2)	676 (9.1)	285 (13.7)	359 (12.1)
Current Cannabis Use (#479)	574 (7.8)	362 (5.0)	180 (2.6)	272 (3.8)	153 (4.8)	98 (2.5)
Amphetamine Use (#599)	312 (4.5)	193 (2.7)	96 (1.5)	177 (2.6)	107 (2.6)	55 (1.4)
Risk Factors – Interpersonal violence and injury						
Physically Attacked (#111)	2,208 (28.6)	1,178 (15.1)	964 (13.2)	779 (10.6)	337 (15.0)	413 (13.2)
Physical Fighting (#130)	2,370 (30.6)	1,582 (20.5)	718 (9.8)	732 (9.9)	383 (20.4)	319 (9.7)
Bullied (#499)	1,824 (24.7)	916 (9.2)	870 (12.9)	535 (7.5)	225 (12.3)	301 (12.5)
Injury (#733)	3,738 (52.1)	2,047 (28.4)	1,606 (23.4)	961 (14.1)	430 (28.4)	502 (23.4)
Risk Factors – Psychological distress						
Psychological Distress (#554)	1,634 (22.3)	679 (12.3)	916 (12.3)	653 (9.1)	215 (9.2)	417 (13.0)

Table 3. Logistic regression results of suicide attempts

Variable	Male		Female	
	Crude Odds Ratio (95% CI)	**Adjusted Odds Ratio (95% CI)**	**Crude Odds Ratio (95% CI)**	**Adjusted Odds Ratio (95% CI)**
Age				
Age in years	1.00 (0.93,1.07)	---	0.99 (0.93,1.05)	---
Risk factors – substance use				
Current Alcohol Use	2.74 (2.27,3.30)***	1.25 (0.98,1.58)	2.73 (2.16,3.44)***	1.78 (1.30,2.42)**
Current Cannabis Use	4.99 (3.79,6.57)***	1.35 (0.78,2.35)	4.28 (3.08,5.98)***	1.98 (1.06,3.67)*
Amphetamine Use	8.38 (5.79, 12.13)***	3.16 (1.28,7.78)*	5.43 (3.89,7.60)***	1.27 (0.53,3.02)
Risk factors – interpersonal violence and injury				
Physically Attacked	3.04 (2.52,3.66)***	1.36 (1.00,1.84)*	3.67 (2.96,4.56)***	2.04 (1.46,2.85)***
Physical Fighting	2.48 (2.00, 3.07)***	1.20 (0.94,1.53)	3.41 (2.94,3.95)***	1.61 (1.24,2.10)**
Bullied	2.51 (2.16,2.91)***	1.87 (1.51,2.32)***	1.98 (1.66, 2.35)***	0.93 (0.77,1.13)
Injury	2.44 (1.94,3.07)***	1.22 (0.90,1.64)	2.16 (1.74,2.70)***	1.38 (1.10,1.75)**
Risk factors – psychological distress				
Psychological Distress	3.10 (2.48,3.87)***	2.69 (2.04,3.54)***	4.05 (3.39,4.83)***	3.02 (2.44,3.73)***

***$p < 0.001$, **$p < 0.01$ *$p < 0.05$; CI: Confidence Interval.

Associations with suicide attempts

In adjusted logistic regression analysis, specifically among males, lifetime amphetamine use (AOR: 3.16, 95% CI: 1.28, 7.78), being physically attacked (AOR: 1.36, 95% CI: 1.00, 1.84), bullied (AOR: 1.87, 95% CI: 1.51, 2.32), and experiencing psychological distress (AOR: 2.69, 95% CI: 2.04, 3.54) were positively associated with suicide attempt in the past 12 months. In addition, in an unadjusted analysis, alcohol use, cannabis use, physical fighting, and injury were positively associated with suicide attempts (see Table 3).

In adjusted logistic regression analysis, specifically among females, current alcohol use (AOR: 1.78, 95% CI: 1.30, 2.42), current cannabis use (AOR: 1.98, 95% CI: 1.06, 3.67), being physically attacked (AOR: 2.04, 95% CI: 1.46, 2.85), being in a physical fight (AOR: 1.61, 95% CI: 1.24, 2.10), injury (AOR: 1.38, 95% CI: 1.10, 1.75), and experiencing psychological distress (AOR: 3.02, 95% CI: 2.44, 3.73) were positively associated with suicide attempt in the past 12 months. In addition, in an unadjusted analysis, among females, being bullied and lifetime amphetamine use was positively associated with suicide attempt (see Table 3).

Discussion

This cross-sectional study investigated the risk factors and gender differences associated with suicide attempts based on the data from school-age adolescents in Bolivia using the 2018 Global School-Based Health Survey. The prevalence of suicide attempts for the past 12 months in the 2012 Bolivia GSHS (20.0%) (20) was similar to the current study (21.4%) but higher than the recorded prevalence of 17.4% among school adolescents in low- to middle-income countries (3). This may be explained in part by Bolivia's economic struggles, ranking one of the lowest in the 2018 Ease of Doing Business report among Latin American and Caribbean countries (21). Their economy continues to face social challenges (22) with 37.2% of the general populace living below the poverty line and the youth unemployment rate at 16.1% (23).

Psychological distress was found to be a risk factor for both sexes, reflecting the poor mental health situation in Bolivia. In Latin American countries, scarcity of resources and sociopolitical obstacles continue to impede access to proper mental healthcare (24). The association between psychological distress (depression) and suicidal behavior was also found in other lower-income countries (17, 25).

With regards to gender differences, findings are consistent with previous literature (17, 18) that more females (25.7%) reported suicide attempts than males (17.5%) in this study, which was higher than female adolescents (16.3%) and male adolescents (9.3%) in Latin American and Caribbean countries (10). For female youths in Bolivia, the findings were similar to previous reports (18) having identified current alcohol use, interpersonal violence (being in a physical fight), and having experienced a serious injury as additional risk factors for suicide attempts. This points to the need for increased awareness and monitoring of substance use as well as gender-based violence and injury prevention among female adolescents in Bolivia.

In contrast, not enough information is available on risk factors for suicide attempts for male youth apart from being threatened on school property (18). This study identified amphetamine use and being bullied as risk factors for suicide attempts among male adolescents in Bolivia. Findings from Latin American studies suggest that being bullied is strongly associated with adolescent suicidal ideation with a plan and at least a single suicide attempt (11). Several culture-specific factors might significantly impact suicidal prevalence and negative health behaviors in Bolivia, including "deeply-rooted gender norms, religious beliefs, and cultural attitudes" (11).

It's important to note that these numbers can be underestimated for sociocultural reasons; a significant portion of suicides are hidden in Bolivia because an individual cannot be given a religious burial if it becomes publicly known that the citizen committed suicide (17).

Study limitations

Owing to the cross-sectional nature of this study, it is only able to report associations and not causative conclusions between variables, and it cannot be generalized beyond school-going adolescents in Bolivia. The data relies on self-reported information which can involve bias regarding their behavior. There was also no physical measurement of height and weight. Lastly, GSHS Bolivia did not control for the rural-urban location of the participating schools.

Conclusion

More than one in five students (one in four females) had attempted suicide in the past 12 months in Bolivia. Several general (both sexes: psychological distress and being physically attacked) and gender-specific factors (males: lifetime amphetamine use, and bullied; females: current alcohol use, current cannabis use, being in a physical fight, and injury) were identified to increase the likelihood of suicide attempt, which can assist in designing suicide prevention in this adolescent population.

Acknowledgments

This paper uses data from the Global School-Based Student Health Survey (GSHS). GSHS is supported by the World Health Organization and the US Centers for Disease Control and Prevention.

References

[1] Lewinsohn PM, Rohde P, Seeley JR. Adolescent suicidal ideation and attempts: Prevalence, risk factors, and clinical implications. Clin Psychol Sci Pract 1996; 3(1):25-46.

[2] World Health Organization. Fact sheet on suicide, 2021. URL: https://www.who.int/news-room/fact-sheets/detail/suicide.

[3] Liu X, Huang Y, Liu Y. Prevalence, distribution, and associated factors of suicide attempts in young adolescents: School-based data from 40 low-income and middle-income countries. PLoS One 2018;13(12):e0207823. doi: 10.1371/journal.pone.0207823.

[4] Mahumud RA, Dawson AJ, Chen W, Biswas T, Keramat SA, Morton RL, et al. The risk and protective factors for suicidal burden among 251 763 school-based adolescents in 77 low- and middle-income to high-income countries: assessing global, regional and national variations. Psychol Med 2022;52(2):379-97. doi: 10.1017/S0033291721002774.

[5] Lagman JG, Gara M, Baweja R, Kim WJ. Correlates of suicide attempts in Filipino youths: An analysis based on the 2015 Global School-Based Student Health Survey. Cureus 2021;13(9):e18100. doi: 10.7759/cureus.18100.

[6] Oppong Asante K, Quarshie EN, Onyeaka HK. Epidemiology of suicidal behaviours amongst school-going adolescents in post-conflict Sierra Leone. J Affect Disord 2021;295:989-96. doi: 10.1016/j.jad.2021.08.147.

[7] Pengpid S, Peltzer K. Prevalence and correlates of past 12-month suicide attempt among in-school adolescents in Guatemala. Psychol Res Behav Manag 2019;12:523-9. doi: 10.2147/PRBM.S212648.

[8] Blum RW, Nelson-Mmari K. The health of young people in a global context. J Adolesc Health 2004;35(5):402-18. doi: 10.1016/j.jadohealth.2003.10.007.

[9] Quinlan-Davidson M, Sanhueza A, Espinosa I, Escamilla-Cejudo JA, Maddaleno M. Suicide among young people in the Americas. J Adolesc Health 2014;54(3):262-8. doi: 10.1016/j.jadohealth.2013.07.012.

[10] Silva AFD, Júnior CASA, Hinnig PF, Lima LRA, Silva DAS. Suicidal behaviors and sedentary lifestyles among adolescents: A cross-sectional epidemiological study in Latin American and Caribbean countries. Clinics (Sao Paulo) 2020;75:e2015. doi: 10.6061/clinics/2020/e2015.

[11] Romo ML, Kelvin EA. Impact of bullying victimization on suicide and negative health behaviors among adolescents in Latin America. Rev Panam Salud Publica 2016;40(5):347-55.

[12] World Bank. GDP current US$ of Bolivia, 2022. URL: https://data.worldbank.org/indicator/NY.GDP.MKTP.CD?locations=BO.

[13] Morgan E. Poverty in Bolivia: Dimensions, political conflict, and strategies. Global Majority E-Journal 2011;2(1):46-59.

[14] Ministry of Health and Sports. National Mental Health Plan 2009–2013. La Paz: Ministry of Health and Sports, 2009.

[15] Jaen-Varas D, Ribeiro WS, Whitfield J, Marı Jde J. Mental health and psychiatric care in Bolivia: What do we know? Int J Ment Health Syst 2014;8:18. doi: 10.1186/1752-4458-8-18.

[16] Garcia M. Mental health in the plurinational State of Bolivia. Int Psychiatry 2011;8(4):88-9.

[17] Jørs E, Christoffersen M, Veirum NH, Aquilar GC, Morant RC, Konradsen F. Suicide attempts and suicides in Bolivia from 2007 to 2012: Pesticides are the preferred method - females try but males commit suicide! Int J Adolesc Med Health 2014;26(3):361-7. doi: 10.1515/ijamh-2013-0309.

[18] Dearden K, De La Cruz N, Crookston B, Novilla L, Clark M. Adolescents at risk: Depression, low academic performance, violence, and alcohol increase Bolivian teenagers' risk of attempted suicide. Int Electron J Health Educ 2005; 8:104-19.

[19] World Health Organization. Global School-based Student Health Survey Bolivia 2018. Fact sheet, 2021. URL: https://extranet.who.int/ncdsmicrodata/index.php/catalog/881/related-materials.

[20] Smith L, Shin JI, Carmichael C, Oh H, Jacob L, López Sánchez GF, et al. Prevalence and correlates of multiple suicide attempts among adolescents aged 12-15 years from 61 countries in Africa, Asia, and the Americas. J Psychiatr Res 2021;144:45-53. doi: 10.1016/j.jpsychires.2021.09.047.

[21] World Bank Group. Doing business, 2018. URL: https://www.doingbusiness.org/content/dam/doingBusiness/media/Annual-Reports/English/DB2018-Full-Report.pdf.

[22] Seelke C. Bolivia: In brief. Congressional Research Service, 2014. URL: https://sgp.fas.org/crs/row/R43473.pdf.

[23] Central Intelligence Agency. The world fact book Bolivia, 2022. URL: https://www.cia.gov/the-world-factbook/countries/bolivia/.

[24] Mascayano F, Irrazabal M, D Emilia W, Vaner SJ, Sapag JC, Alvarado R, et al. Suicide in Latin America: a growing public health issue. Rev Fac Cien Med Univ Nac Cordoba 2015;72(4):295-303.

[25] Lee H, Lee EY, Greene B, Shin YJ. Psychological distress among adolescents in Laos, Mongolia, Nepal, and Sri Lanka. Asian Nurs Res (Korean Soc Nurs Sci) 2019;13(2):147-53. doi: 10.1016/j.anr.2019.04.001.

Section two: Acknowledgements

Chapter 17

About the editor

Joav Merrick, MD, MMedSci, DMSc, born and educated in Denmark is professor of pediatrics, Division of Pediatrics, Hadassah Hebrew University Medical Center, Mt Scopus Campus, Jerusalem, Israel and Kentucky Children's Hospital, University of Kentucky, Lexington, Kentucky United States and professor of public health at the Center for Healthy Development, School of Public Health, Georgia State University, Atlanta, United States, the former medical director of the Health Services, Division for Intellectual and Developmental Disabilities, Ministry of Social Affairs and Social Services, Jerusalem, the founder and director of the National Institute of Child Health and Human Development in Israel. Numerous publications in the field of pediatrics, child health and human development, rehabilitation, intellectual disability, disability, health, welfare, abuse, advocacy, quality of life and prevention. Received the Peter Sabroe Child Award for outstanding work on behalf of Danish Children in 1985 and the International LEGO-Prize ("The Children's Nobel Prize") for an extraordinary contribution towards improvement in child welfare and well-being in 1987 and in 2017 appointed a Kentucky Colonel by the Commonwealth of Kentucky, the highest honor the governor can bestow to a person. Email: jmerrick@zahav.net.il.

Chapter 18

About the National Institute of Child Health and Human Development in Israel

The National Institute of Child Health and Human Development (NICHD) in Israel was established in 1998 as a virtual institute under the auspices of the Medical Director, Ministry of Social Affairs and Social Services in order to function as the research arm for the Office of the Medical Director. In 1998 the National Council for Child Health and Pediatrics, Ministry of Health and in 1999 the Director General and Deputy Director General of the Ministry of Health endorsed the establishment of the NICHD.

Mission

The mission of a National Institute for Child Health and Human Development in Israel is to provide an academic focal point for the scholarly interdisciplinary study of child life, health, public health, welfare, disability, rehabilitation, intellectual disability and related aspects of human development. This mission includes research, teaching, clinical work, information and public service activities in the field of child health and human development.

Service and academic activities

Over the years many activities became focused in the south of Israel due to collaboration with various professionals at the Faculty of Health Sciences (FOHS) at the Ben Gurion University of the Negev (BGU). Since 2000 an affiliation with the Zusman Child Development Center at the Pediatric Division of Soroka University Medical Center has resulted in collaboration around the establishment of the Down Syndrome Clinic at that center. In 2002 a full course on "Disability" was established at the Recanati School for Allied Professions in the Community, FOHS, BGU and in 2005 collaboration was started with the Primary Care Unit of the faculty and disability became part of the master of public health course on "Children and society". In the academic year 2005-2006 a one semester course on "Aging with disability" was started as part of the master of science program in gerontology in our collaboration with the Center for Multidisciplinary Research in Aging. In 2010 collaborations with the Division of Pediatrics, Hadassah Hebrew University Medical Center, Jerusalem, Israel around the National Down Syndrome Center and teaching students and residents about intellectual and developmental disabilities as part of their training at this campus.

Research activities

The affiliated staff have over the years published work from projects and research activities in this national and international collaboration. In the year 2000 the International Journal of Adolescent Medicine and Health and in 2005 the International Journal on Disability and Human Development of De Gruyter Publishing House (Berlin and New York) were affiliated with the National Institute of Child Health and Human Development. From 2008 also the International Journal of Child Health and Human Development (Nova Science, New York), the International Journal of Child and Adolescent Health (Nova Science) and the Journal of Pain Management (Nova Science) affiliated and from 2009 the International Public Health Journal (Nova Science) and Journal of Alternative Medicine Research (Nova Science). All peer-reviewed international journals.

National collaborations

Nationally the NICHD works in collaboration with the Faculty of Health Sciences, Ben Gurion University of the Negev; Department of Physical Therapy, Sackler School of Medicine, Tel Aviv University; Autism Center, Assaf HaRofeh Medical Center; National Rett and PKU Centers at Chaim Sheba Medical Center, Tel HaShomer; Department of Physiotherapy, Haifa University; Department of Education, Bar Ilan University, Ramat Gan, Faculty of Social Sciences and Health Sciences; College of Judea and Samaria in Ariel and in 2011 affiliation with Center for Pediatric Chronic Diseases and

National Center for Down Syndrome, Department of Pediatrics, Hadassah Hebrew University Medical Center, Mount Scopus Campus, Jerusalem.

International collaborations

Internationally with the Department of Disability and Human Development, College of Applied Health Sciences, University of Illinois at Chicago; Strong Center for Developmental Disabilities, Golisano Children's Hospital at Strong, University of Rochester School of Medicine and Dentistry, New York; Centre on Intellectual Disabilities, University of Albany, New York; Centre for Chronic Disease Prevention and Control, Health Canada, Ottawa; Chandler Medical Center and Children's Hospital, Kentucky Children's Hospital, Section of Adolescent Medicine, University of Kentucky, Lexington; Chronic Disease Prevention and Control Research Center, Baylor College of Medicine, Houston, Texas; Division of Neuroscience, Department of Psychiatry, Columbia University, New York; Institute for the Study of Disadvantage and Disability, Atlanta; Center for Autism and Related Disorders, Department Psychiatry, Children's Hospital Boston, Boston; Department of Pediatric and Adolescent Medicine, Western Michigan University Homer Stryker MD School of Medicine, Kalamazoo, Michigan, United States; Department of Paediatrics, Child Health and Adolescent Medicine, Children's Hospital at Westmead, Westmead, Australia; International Centre for the Study of Occupational and Mental Health, Düsseldorf, Germany; Centre for Advanced Studies in Nursing, Department of General Practice and Primary Care, University of Aberdeen, Aberdeen, United Kingdom; Quality of Life Research Center, Copenhagen, Denmark; Nordic School of Public Health, Gottenburg, Sweden, Scandinavian Institute of Quality of Working Life, Oslo, Norway; The Department of Applied Social Sciences (APSS) of The Hong Kong Polytechnic University Hong Kong.

Targets

Our focus is on research, international collaborations, clinical work, teaching and policy in health, disability and human development and to establish the NICHD as a permanent institute in Israel in order to conduct model research and policy.

Contact

Professor Joav Merrick, MD, MMedSci, DMSc
Director, National Institute of Child Health and Human Development,
Jerusalem, Israel. E-mail: jmerrick@zahav.net.il

Section three: Index

Index

A

B

C

D

L

M

N

O

P

R

S

T

U

W

Y